CRQs and SBAs for the Final FRCA:
questions and detailed answers

CRQs and SBAs for the Final FRCA: questions and detailed answers

D. Sumner
MBBS, BSc, FRCA
Registrar in Anaesthetics and Intensive Care

C. Allen
MBBS, BA
Fellow in Regional Anaesthesia

A. Feneley
MBBS, BSc, FRCA
Trauma Anaesthesia Fellow

M. Raithatha
MBBS, BSc, FRCA
Senior Trainee in Anaesthetics

Scion

A CIP catalogue record for this book is available from the British Library.

Scion Publishing Limited
The Old Hayloft, Vantage Business Park, Bloxham Road, Banbury OX16 9UX, UK
www.scionpublishing.com

Important Note from the Publisher
The information contained within this book was obtained by Scion Publishing Ltd from sources believed by us to be reliable. However, while every effort has been made to ensure its accuracy, no responsibility for loss or injury whatsoever occasioned to any person acting or refraining from action as a result of information contained herein can be accepted by the authors or publishers.

Readers are reminded that medicine is a constantly evolving science and while the authors and publishers have ensured that all dosages, applications and practices are based on current indications, there may be specific practices which differ between communities. You should always follow the guidelines laid down by the manufacturers of specific products and the relevant authorities in the country in which you are practising.

Although every effort has been made to ensure that all owners of copyright material have been acknowledged in this publication, we would be pleased to acknowledge in subsequent reprints or editions any omissions brought to our attention.

Registered names, trademarks, etc. used in this book, even when not marked as such, are not to be considered unprotected by law.

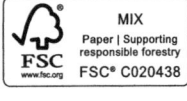
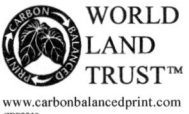

www.carbonbalancedprint.com
CBP2250

Typeset by Medlar Publishing Solutions Pvt Ltd, India
Printed in the UK by Hobbs the Printers Ltd

Last digit is the print number: 10 9 8 7 6 5 4

Contents

About the authors

Dan Sumner MBBS BSc (Hons) FRCA RCPathMe is a dual Anaesthetic and Intensive care registrar in the Kent, Surrey and Sussex School of Anaesthesia. He has a special interest in high-risk perioperative care and invasive ventilation. He has taught on multiple anaesthetic viva courses for both the primary and final FRCA as well as being the founder of 'smash finals', a national teaching programme for medical school final exams. He also acts as a reviewer for *BMJ Case Reports*.

Catherine Allen MBBS BA (Hons) is an Anaesthetic registrar in the Kent, Surrey and Sussex School of Anaesthesia. She has a special interest in simulation and medical education as well as regional anaesthesia, having recently completed a fellowship post in regional anaesthesia.

Andrew Feneley MBBS BSc (Hons) PGCert FRCA MAcadMEd is an Anaesthetic registrar in the South East London School of Anaesthesia. He has special interests in paediatric anaesthesia, trauma and medical education. As well as hospital-based practice, Andrew is also a trackside doctor at motorsport events in the UK and internationally.

Mehul Raithatha MBBS BSc (Hons) FRCA is an Anaesthetic registrar in the East of England School of Anaesthesia. His special interests include both acute and chronic pain, including invasive pain-related procedures, regional anaesthesia and teaching; having designed a regional teaching programme in the east of England.

Preface

The award of the Fellowship of the Royal College of Anaesthetists has always been one of the most prestigious awards in clinical medicine. Candidates sitting the exam spend hours of blood, sweat and sometimes tears in pursuit of a pass.

Anaesthesia is a dynamic field and so is the exam, with the structure of the exam undergoing significant change over the last few years. Traditionally the exam comprised Short Answer Questions (essay-style questions) and multiple choice (true/false) questions. This has changed to more structured Constructed Response Questions (CRQs) and, more recently, Single Best Answer questions replacing multiple choice.

On top of this, the anaesthetic training curriculum has recently undergone a complete overhaul. Whilst the core knowledge underpinning the training in anaesthesia has largely remained the same, the timepoints and expected milestones have somewhat changed. It is not uncommon for a candidate to sit their exams before completing some of the specialist modules on which the questions are based.

We have written this book to reflect the new style of exams and to be able to sit each practice paper as a timed mock exam, should a candidate wish, as well as give a helpful overview of some of the topics – especially those considered specialist.

Overall, we hope this will help anyone sitting their final FRCA prepare for the exam and go to their sitting with as much practice as possible.

D. Sumner
C. Allen
A. Feneley
M. Raithatha

Acknowledgements

The authors would like to thank Dr Philip Blackie MBBS FRCA FFICM EDIC RCPathME DLM, Consultant anaesthetist, for kindly editing a significant part of the SBA section of this book.

DS: To Cathy for allowing me the time to write this book, and to Jonny and Lily for not allowing me the time to write this book.

CA: I'd like to thank Dan for his continued support, Jonny and Lily for the ongoing distraction, my parents and all of the people who have taught me what I know.

AF: To Lizzie, Charlotte, my parents and the rest of my family for their support and patience.

MR: To my parents for their guidance, to my brother Rishi for educating me constantly, and to my wife Sneha for her endless patience, encouragement and support.

Practice Paper 1

CRQ 1: The pharmacokinetics of sepsis

Sepsis is one of the most common reasons for inpatient morbidity and mortality in the UK.

a Define sepsis. (2 marks)

i. ....

ii. ....

b What underlying pathological features of sepsis contribute to end organ damage? (3 marks)

i. ....

ii. ....

iii. ....

c Outline how the following pharmacokinetic principles would be altered in a patient with **severe sepsis**.

Absorption (4 marks)

i. ....

ii. ....

iii. ....

iv. ....

Distribution (3 marks)

i. ....

ii. ....

iii. ....

Metabolism (1 mark)

i. ....

Elimination (1 mark)

i. ....

d Explain the pharmacokinetics of propofol administration in patients with severe sepsis. (3 marks)

i. ....

ii. ....

iii. ....

e With prolonged sepsis, the doses of some vasoactive substances may need increasing to maintain the same degree of responsiveness. Explain the pharmacological mechanism for this. (3 marks)

i. ....

ii. ....

iii. ....

CRQ 2: Major obstetric haemorrhage

A 31-year-old woman presents to the hospital's anaesthetic antenatal clinic. She is a Jehovah's Witness and has a low-lying placenta. She has not had any previous surgeries, and is otherwise fit and well. She has previously stated that she would not accept a blood transfusion.

a List three haematological changes that occur in pregnancy. (3 marks)

i. ....

ii. ....

iii. ....

b What two pre-operative interventions and two intra-operative interventions can be used to prevent blood loss during this surgery? (4 marks)

i. Pre-op ....

ii. Pre-op ....

iii. Intra-op ....

iv. Intra-op ....

c List three advantages and three disadvantages of intra-operative cell salvage use. (6 marks)

i. Advantage ....

ii. Advantage ....

iii. Advantage ....

i. Disadvantage ....

ii. Disadvantage ....

iii. Disadvantage ....

d List one absolute contraindication (as per the Intensive Care Society standard practice) for the use of intra-operative cell salvage. (1 mark)

i. ....

The patient presents at 38 weeks' gestation for an elective caesarean section. During the procedure the patient becomes tachycardic and hypotensive. The surgical team states there has been 2 litres of blood loss so far. A sample is taken for analysis by thromboelastography.

e Label the sections of the diagram (annotated as 1–5), and explain how each labelled part of the trace relates to blood clot formation. (5 marks)

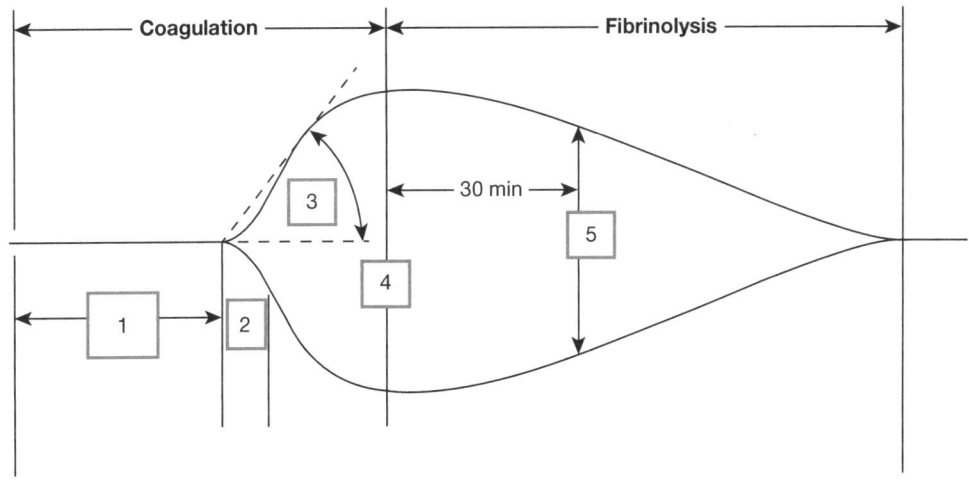

1. ....

2. ....

3. ....

4. ....

5. ....

f The patient continues to bleed and the surgeons are considering performing a hysterectomy. Your colleague states that based on the TEG trace, the patient is likely to be in early DIC. Describe how the TEG trace is altered in early DIC. (1 mark)

i. ....

CRQ 3:   Head trauma management

A 46-year-old patient is admitted to the emergency department following a road traffic collision (RTC). He has sustained a head injury.

a List six indications for intubation in patients with head trauma.   (6 marks)

i. ....

ii. ....

iii. ....

iv. ....

v. ....

vi. ....

b List four indications for maintaining cervical spine immobilisation in patients who have sustained a head injury (before imaging has been obtained).   (4 marks)

i. ....

ii. ....

iii. ....

iv. ....

c State one advantage (1 mark) and one disadvantage (1 mark) for using ketamine, rather than propofol, for induction of anaesthesia in the head-injured patient.

i. Advantage ....

i. Disadvantage ....

d What is secondary traumatic brain injury (1 mark), and over what timeframe (1 mark) does it occur?

i. ....

ii. Timeframe ....

e What is the target cerebral perfusion pressure (CPP) in mmHg in patients
with a head injury?   (1 mark)

i. ....

f Describe, with doses where applicable, five strategies to control raised
intracranial pressure (ICP).   (5 marks)

i. ....

ii. ....

iii. ....

iv. ....

v. ....

CRQ 4: Awake fibre-optic intubation

A 69-year-old patient presents for an elective right hemi-colectomy for colon cancer. Her past medical history includes rheumatoid arthritis, with limited neck movement. Upon review of her previous anaesthetic charts you notice she has a 'known difficult airway'.

a List two indications (1 mark) and four contraindications (2 marks) for awake fibre-optic intubation.

  i. **Indication** ....

  ii. **Indication** ....

  i. **Contraindication** ....

  ii. **Contraindication** ....

  iii. **Contraindication** ....

  iv. **Contraindication** ....

b Name six terminal nerves that have to be blocked, via direct injection or topicalisation, to provide anaesthesia for an awake fibre-optic intubation. (6 marks)

  i. ....

  ii. ....

  iii. ....

  iv. ....

  v. ....

  vi. ....

c What is the maximum dose of lidocaine that can be used for topicalisation of the airway? (1 mark)

  i. ....

d What is the quantity of lidocaine contained within the co-phenylcaine spray used for nasal airway topicalisation? (1 mark)

i. ....

e According to the Difficult Airway Society (DAS) awake fibre-optic guidelines (2020), what are the two options available for sedation? (2 marks)

i. ....

ii. ....

f After insertion of the endotracheal tube, what methods can be used to ensure correct tube placement? (2 marks)

i. ....

ii. ....

g List five complications of an awake fibre-optic intubation. (5 marks)

i. ....

ii. ....

iii. ....

iv. ....

v. ....

CRQ 5: Trigeminal neuralgia

A 55-year-old woman presents to the pain clinic with new onset facial pain. She was referred by her GP, who has ruled out migraines, and she has had a CT head that demonstrates no intracranial pathology. You suspect she has trigeminal neuralgia.

a List five risk factors for developing trigeminal neuralgia. (5 marks)

i. ....

ii. ....

iii. ....

iv. ....

v. ....

b In the table below, list the foramina through which the divisions of the trigeminal nerve pass through the base of the skull. (3 marks)

Division of the trigeminal nerve (CN V)	Base of skull foramen through which it passes
V1 (ophthalmic)	i. ....
V2 (maxillary)	ii. ....
V3 (mandibular)	iii. ....

c List three of the five diagnostic criteria based on the clinical characteristics of trigeminal neuralgia. (3 marks)

i. ....

ii. ....

iii. ....

d For each of the following pharmacological agents, document the class of the drug and the receptor at which they act. If a drug acts at more than one receptor, list only one. (6 marks)

Carbamazepine

  i. Class ....

 ii. Receptor ....

Gabapentin

  i. Class ....

 ii. Receptor ....

Amitriptyline

  i. Class ....

 ii. Receptor ....

e List three options for the surgical management of trigeminal neuralgia. (3 marks)

   i. ....

  ii. ....

 iii. ....

CRQ 6: Congenital diaphragmatic hernia

You have been called to assist in the delivery suite, as the neonatologists are managing a neonate in distress. The neonate was born at term via an uncomplicated vaginal delivery in the midwifery-led care area, due to the mother being low risk. The neonatologists suspect that the baby has a previously undiagnosed congenital diaphragmatic hernia (CDH).

a List two signs that may be seen in a baby with CDH. (2 marks)

i. ....

ii. ....

b What will a plain chest radiograph demonstrate in CDH? (1 mark)

i. ....

c 10% of patients with CDH will have an associated genetic or chromosomal abnormality. Name two of these conditions. (2 marks)

i. ....

ii. ....

d CDH is often associated with structural abnormalities of the heart. List two of the most common cardiac anatomical abnormalities seen in patients with CDH. (2 marks)

i. ....

ii. ....

e List four postnatal features that would suggest a poor prognosis for this neonate. (4 marks)

i. ....

ii. ....

iii. ....

iv. ....

f Outline the essential steps in the medical management of CDH – other than pharmacological therapy – including which investigation(s) should be ordered immediately after delivery. (3 marks)

....

....

....

g List three types of pharmacological therapy that would be useful, and state why. (3 marks)

  i. ....

  ii. ....

  iii. ....

A decision is made to proceed with surgical correction of the defect.

h What physiological parameters should be achieved prior to surgery, as per the CDH Euro-Consortium guidelines? (3 marks)

  i. ....

  ii. ....

  iii. ....

CRQ 7: Bone cement implantation syndrome

A 79-year-old woman is due to undergo an emergency hemi-arthroplasty following a fall at home. She has a background of ischaemic heart disease with a previous coronary artery bypass graft, COPD, current smoker, and has had a recent diagnosis of non-small cell lung cancer.

She receives a spinal anaesthetic and sedation with propofol (TCI). The surgeons wish to use bone cement to facilitate joint fixation.

a What is the main constituent of bone cement? (1 mark)

i. ....

b List two advantages of using bone cement in hemi-arthoplasties. (2 marks)

i. ....

ii. ....

The operating surgeon wishes to use a bone cement impregnated with antibiotics.

c List two antibiotics that can be used within bone cement. (2 marks)

i. ....

ii. ....

d List three disadvantages of using antibiotic-containing bone cement, compared to bone cement without antibiotics. (3 marks)

i. ....

ii. ....

iii. ....

During the procedure the patient becomes agitated despite propofol sedation, hypoxic and tachycardic. The blood pressure cuff cycles but a reading is not displayed. You suspect bone cement implantation syndrome (BCIS).

e   List two patient factors and two surgical factors that predispose to BCIS.   (4 marks)

   i. Patient factor ....

 ii. Patient factor...

   i. Surgical factor ....

 ii. Surgical factor...

f   Describe the grades of BCIS in terms of their severity.   (3 marks)

   i. Grade I ....

 ii. Grade II ....

iii. Grade III ....

g   List and describe the two proposed aetiological models for the development of BCIS, and their pathophysiological mechanism.   (2 marks)

   i. ....

 ii. ....

h   Describe three ways in which BCIS can be prevented peri-operatively by the operating surgeon, excluding the use of an uncemented prosthesis.   (3 marks)

   i. ....

 ii. ....

iii. ....

CRQ 8:   Burns

A patient has arrived at the accident and emergency department having been involved in a house fire, caused by a faulty electrical circuit. The patient was found unconscious in the living room – where the fire started – but regained consciousness when extracted by the fire service. He has visible burns across both arms and his entire chest. His head and neck have been spared. He is estimated to weigh around 90kg.

a Calculate the total volume of fluid that the patient will require in the first 24 hours following the burn injury, and duration over which the fluids will be infused. (Please show working)   (4 marks)

....

....

....

....

b What are the indications for intubation in a patient brought to hospital with burns?   (5 marks)

i.   ....

ii.   ....

iii.   ....

iv.   ....

v.   ....

c What clinical, pharmacological and practical factors should be considered when intubating the patient?   (3 marks)

i.   ....

ii.   ....

iii.   ....

d When should the patient be discussed with the on-call burns consultant, or transferred to a regional burns centre? (5 marks)

i. ....

ii. ....

iii. ....

iv. ....

v. ....

e What are the possible early (<48 hours) complications of burns? (3 marks)

i. ....

ii. ....

iii. ....

CRQ 9:   Intra-aortic balloon pump

A 48-year-old patient returns from the cardiothoracic theatre with an intra-aortic balloon pump *in situ*. You have been asked to review them post-operatively.

---

a | What is the primary physiological goal of an intra-aortic balloon pump (IABP)?

(2 marks)

....

....

b | List four indications for the insertion of an IABP.

(2 marks)

i. ....

ii. ....

iii. ....

iv. ....

c | List three absolute contraindications for the insertion of an IABP.

(3 marks)

i. ....

ii. ....

iii. ....

d | List the haemodynamic effects of the IABP with regard to systolic/diastolic pressure, afterload/preload, wall tension, cardiac output and coronary blood flow, on the following areas.

(4 marks)

i. **Aorta** ....

ii. **Left ventricle** ....

iii. **Heart** ....

iv. **Blood flow** ....

e State the gas used to insufflate the balloon of an IABP, and explain the rationale behind its use. (2 marks)

....

....

f Label the following graphical representation of the arterial trace with an IABP *in situ*. (4 marks)

1. ....

2. ....

3. ....

4. ....

g What is the equation for coronary perfusion pressure? (1 mark)

....

h Explain how the patient can be weaned from an IABP to resume normal physiological cardiac function. (2 marks)

....

....

CRQ 10: Awareness

You have been asked to see a patient in distress, whom you had anaesthetised a day ago for a laparoscopic hysterectomy. You remember that the procedure and anaesthetic had no complications. The patient says she was aware of what was going on throughout the procedure and wants to know why this has happened.

a What are the two types of awareness and what are their respective characteristics?

(2 marks)

i. ....

ii. ....

b What is the incidence of awareness in the following? (3 marks)

i. **Anaesthetic with neuromuscular blocker** ....

ii. **Anaesthetic without neuromuscular blocker** ....

iii. **All general anaesthetics** ....

c List **six** clinical signs that may indicate a patient could be inadvertently aware under anaesthesia. (3 marks)

i. ....

ii. ....

iii. ....

d List four methods to monitor depth of anaesthesia. (4 marks)

i. ....

ii. ....

iii. ....

iv. ....

e   Other than the use of neuromuscular blockers, list five risk factors for developing awareness under anaesthesia.   (5 marks)

i. ....

ii. ....

iii. ....

iv. ....

v. ....

f   According to the NAP5 awareness support pathway, what three support mechanisms or interventions should be offered to a patient who has suspected awareness?   (3 marks)

i. ....

ii. ....

iii. ....

CRQ 11: Autism spectrum disorder

You are the anaesthetist for a day surgery dental list in paediatrics. The list includes a 16-year-old girl with autism spectrum disorder (ASD) who has not had any previous medical procedures. The patient's parents are very anxious regarding their daughter's care and have asked for more information on what to expect.

a What are the triad of features that characterise autism spectrum disorder? (3 marks)

i. ....

ii. ....

iii. ....

b List four challenges that may be faced when undertaking a pre-operative assessment in this patient. (4 marks)

i. ....

ii. ....

iii. ....

iv. ....

c Prior to the surgery, how can the pre-assessment and admissions process (up to entering the anaesthetic room) be streamlined to facilitate the least amount of distress for the patient? (4 marks)

i. ....

ii. ....

iii. ....

iv. ....

d List four options for pre-medicating the patient (with doses) to help facilitate the surgery. (4 marks)

i. ....

ii. ....

iii. ....

iv. ....

e What possible issues may need to be overcome in the post-operative period? (3 marks)

i. ....

ii. ....

iii. ....

f List two possible ways in which you could communicate with the patient in the post-operative period. (2 marks)

i. ....

ii. ....

CRQ 12: Serotonin syndrome

You are assessing a patient prior to a routine general surgical inguinal hernia repair. The patient takes antidepressant medication and has been doing some research about their anaesthetic prior to attending hospital. They have been reading about the condition serotonin syndrome and wish to know more.

---

a What are the triad of symptoms/features of serotonin syndrome? (3 marks)

i. ....

ii. ....

iii. ....

b Other than the symptoms, what other patient-related factor must be present to make a diagnosis of serotonin syndrome? (1 mark)

....

c What laboratory tests would be helpful in making a diagnosis of serotonin syndrome? (3 marks)

i. ....

ii. ....

iii. ....

d List four differentials for serotonin syndrome. (4 marks)

i. ....

ii. ....

iii. ....

iv. ....

e Where in the brain is serotonin synthesised? (1 mark)
List three other locations within the CNS, or body, where it is found. (3 marks)

i. Synthesised ....

i. Location ....

ii. Location ....

iii. Location ....

f How many serotonin receptor classes are found within the body? (1 mark)

....

g Complete the table with examples of a drug, or drug class, that has the
following effects on serotonin. (4 marks)

Serotonin synthesis	L-tryptophan
Enhanced serotonin release	i. ....
Serotonin reuptake inhibition	ii. ....
Serotonin metabolism	iii. ....
Direct agonist	iv. ....

SBA 1:

A 30-year-old 7 day post-partum woman presents to the labour ward with a worsening headache over the last 4 days. The headache is 10/10 in severity and particularly feels like pressure behind both eyes, with some blurred vision. She had an uneventful caesarean section, but was found to be anaemic post-operatively, requiring transfusion of 1 unit packed red cells. She is otherwise fit and well.

What would be the most appropriate investigation for this patient?

A. No further investigation needed – conservative management only
B. No further investigation needed – book patient for epidural blood patch
C. CT head
D. CT venogram of head
E. MRI brain

SBA 2:

Which of these conditions presents the highest risk for malignant hyperthermia under anaesthesia?

A. Myasthenia gravis
B. Duchenne muscular dystrophy
C. Guillain–Barré syndrome
D. Central core myopathy
E. Muscular dystrophy

SBA 3:

Which of the following is an absolute indication for one-lung ventilation?

A. Pneumonectomy
B. Lung volume reduction surgery
C. Upper lobectomy
D. Mediastinal mass reduction
E. Single lung lavage in cystic fibrosis

SBA 4:

An 18-year-old patient presents for an ulnar ORIF following a motorbike accident 3 days prior. He is requesting a regional anaesthetic technique rather than a general anaesthetic technique.

What is the most appropriate regional anaesthetic block to perform on this patient?

A. Interscalene block
B. Supraclavicular block
C. Infraclavicular block
D. Axillary block
E. Direct block of the ulnar nerve

SBA 5:

Which of the following is not true regarding the anatomy of the autonomic nervous system?

A. Preganglionic fibres in the sympathetic nervous system originate from cell bodies in the grey matter of the lateral horn of the spinal cord
B. The paravertebral sympathetic chain is divided into four parts
C. The thoracic paravertebral sympathetic chain consists of ganglia from T1–T7
D. Cranial parasympathetic fibres arise from the 3rd, 7th, 9th and 10th cranial nerves
E. Preganglionic fibres are myelinated and post-ganglionic fibres are unmyelinated, in both the sympathetic and parasympathetic nervous systems

SBA 6:

A 56-year-old woman is undergoing a right-sided mastectomy and sentinel lymph node biopsy following a diagnosis of breast cancer. She has no other past medical history and has previously had a general anaesthetic for a hysteroscopy without any complications. She is intubated and ventilated and the surgical time-out has been performed. The surgeons inject patent blue dye and the patient becomes tachycardic at a rate of 150bpm and hypotensive to 48/23mmHg.

What is the immediate management of the patient?

A. IV adrenaline 50mcg
B. IM adrenaline 0.5mg
C. Start 500ml NaCl 0.9% IV
D. Hydrocortisone 100mg IV
E. Commence CPR

SBA 7:

A 56-year-old man is transferred to the intensive care unit following an elective AAA repair. He has a history of heavy smoking and hypertension but is otherwise well. A chest X-ray performed following the procedure to check the position of an internal jugular line shows a pneumothorax, measuring 1.5cm at the level of the hilum.

What is the management required for this pneumothorax?

A. Apply 100% O_2 and repeat chest X-ray in 24 hours
B. Aspirate with 16–18G cannula
C. Insertion of 8–14Fr Seldinger chest drain
D. Insertion of surgical chest drain
E. Observation only

SBA 8:

A 4-week-old baby boy presents with recurrent projectile vomiting after feeding. He has been diagnosed with pyloric stenosis and is scheduled to undergo a pyloromyotomy.

Which of the following factors makes pyloric stenosis more likely?

A. Female gender
B. White ethnicity
C. Pre-term delivery
D. Maternal *Helicobacter pylori* infection
E. Forceps delivery

SBA 9:

A 79-year-old man with severe vascular disease has been listed for a right below-knee amputation. He has previously had a below-knee amputation of his left leg and recalls severe stump pain, and continues to have phantom limb pain.

What would be the optimum pain relief strategy to prevent phantom limb pain after this operation?

A. Femoral and popliteal block with perineural catheters inserted and post-operative infusion of local anaesthetic
B. Epidural anaesthesia with bupivacaine and fentanyl
C. IV lidocaine infusion started intra-operatively and continued post-operatively
D. PCA morphine
E. Spinal anaesthesia with diamorphine and bupivacaine

SBA 10:

A 53-year-old woman is due to undergo DIEP flap breast reconstruction, 7 months after her original mastectomy for breast cancer.

Which of the following is an absolute contraindication to undergoing free-flap surgery?

A. Age >70
B. Smoking
C. Obesity
D. Sickle cell trait
E. Polycythaemia rubra vera

SBA 11:

A neonate born at term is noted to have difficulty clearing secretions, with repeated episodes of choking and coughing. The neonatologists have diagnosed oesophageal atresia. The neonate has been prepared for surgery with the insertion of a Replogle tube, prophylactic antibiotics and IV fluids. The baby proceeds to surgery and is transferred to the paediatric intensive care unit following the successful procedure.

What is the most common early complication of this type of surgery that the baby may suffer from?

A. Post-operative chest infection
B. Anastomotic leak
C. Tracheomalacia
D. Oesophageal stricture
E. Gastro-oesophageal reflux

SBA 12:

Which of the following local anaesthetics matches the correct pKa?

A. Lidocaine – 7.4
B. Bupivacaine – 7.8
C. Prilocaine – 7.0
D. Ropivacaine – 8.1
E. Cocaine – 8.0

SBA 13:

A 30-year-old G2P1 has presented to the labour ward following a successful induction of labour. She is now in established labour and would like an epidural for pain relief. An epidural is sited with some difficulty and she is given a test dose of 12ml of low dose mix (0.125% levobupivacaine and 1mcg/ml fentanyl). Within the first 2 minutes she has arm weakness and difficulty in breathing, and begins to have fluctuating consciousness. She has continuous CTG monitoring and the midwives state that the CTG is normal. She has 500ml of fluid rapidly infused and 100% oxygen is applied.

What is the next step in the patient's immediate management?

A. Immediate intubation and ventilation with CAT 1 caesarean section
B. Immediate intubation and ventilation and monitor patient in the operating theatre
C. Removal of epidural catheter and monitor the patient
D. Immediate bolus then infusion of intralipid
E. Place patient in left lateral and give further bolus of fluid

SBA 14:

A 32-year-old woman is due to be anaesthetised for an emergency appendicectomy.

Which of the following is the most significant predictor of difficult face mask ventilation?

A. Obesity
B. Edentulous
C. Mallampati 4
D. Snorer
E. Neck irradiation

SBA 15:

Which of the following is the strongest risk factor for a peri-procedural stroke in patients with coexisting atrial fibrillation?

A. Tissue aortic valve
B. $CHADS_2$ score >3
C. History of TIA – several years ago
D. TIA 4 years previously
E. Stroke 16 years previously

SBA 16:

A 24-year-old presents with neuropathic left leg pain following a crush injury from an RTC.

The following are first-line treatments for neuropathic pain except:

A. Amitriptyline
B. Duloxetine
C. Gabapentin
D. Pregabalin
E. Carbamazepine

SBA 17:

A 5-year-old presents to A&E with a 3-day history of general malaise and lethargy. Over the last 4 hours the child has become less responsive and febrile. On examination there is a widespread purpuric rash, with hypotension and tachycardia. The paediatric team has given a total of 720ml of fluid with no response.

What is the next step in this patient's management?

A. Further fluid bolus 20ml/kg
B. Start IV dopamine 10mcg/kg/min
C. Start central noradrenaline 0.1mcg/kg/min
D. Immediate intubation and ventilation
E. Start IV phenylephrine 0.5mg/min

SBA 18:

A 32-year-old patient with high grade lymphoma has received his first round of chemotherapy on the haematology ward. He has become febrile and his urgent blood tests are as follows: potassium 6.2mmol/L (previously 4.4), creatinine 400mg/dL (previously 74) and pH 7.21 on VBG.

What is the most appropriate choice of management for this patient?

A. Immediate CVVHF
B. IV rasburicase
C. IV allopurinol
D. Forced alkaline diuresis
E. IV sodium bicarbonate

SBA 19:

A 45-year-old man presents to hospital with intermittent tachycardia, tremor and abdominal pain. A diagnosis of phaeochromocytoma is made and the patient is listed for laparoscopic resection of his adrenal mass.

Which of the following is not a risk factor for intraoperative haemodynamic instability?

A. Large tumour size
B. High pre-operative plasma noradrenaline level
C. Pre-induction mean arterial pressure of >100mmHg
D. Open surgery (vs. laparoscopic surgery)
E. Postural drop after commencement of alpha blockade

SBA 20:

Which of the following is a correct description of phase III of the Valsalva manoeuvre?

A. Baroreceptor reflex activation causes a vasoconstriction and tachycardia, trending BP towards normal
B. Intrathoracic pressure is suddenly released and associated pooling of blood in pulmonary vessels causes a drop in BP
C. Blood is expelled from the thoracic vessels by an increase in intrathoracic pressure
D. Reduction in venous return due to increase in intrathoracic pressure
E. Overshoot in BP as compensatory mechanisms operate

SBA 21:

A 60-year-old woman listed for elective shoulder replacement is concerned about post-operative pain. You consent her for a combination of general anaesthetic with opiates and regional blockade. She has an uneventful operation and is extubated in theatre before transfer to the post-operative care unit. You are called 20 minutes later as she is feeling short of breath and having difficulty taking deep breaths. Her oxygen saturations are 96% on a 15L non-rebreathe mask.

What is the most likely cause of her shortness of breath?

A. Inadequate reversal
B. Post-operative anxiety
C. Opiate toxicity
D. Phrenic nerve palsy
E. Intra-operative MI

SBA 22:

A 65-year-old patient presents for routine hernia surgery. He has a history of cardiac arrest in the past which was secondary to myocardial infarction. Following the cardiac arrest he had an implantable cardiac device (ICD) inserted.

When is the optimal time for this to be deactivated peri-operatively?

A. Pre-operatively in day surgery ward
B. In the anaesthetic room prior to induction
C. In the anaesthetic room post induction
D. In the operating theatre before incision
E. The ICD does not need to be deactivated

SBA 23:

A 46-year-old patient presents for washout and debridement of an infected peri-anal abscess. They have been paraplegic since being in a car accident 26 years prior, which resulted in complete transection of the spinal cord at level T6. On examination, they have no sensation below the level of the lesion and have had multiple anaesthetics in the past without any issue within the last 10 years. They have no other coexisting medical conditions.

Regarding anaesthetic requirements, what is the most appropriate option?

A. General anaesthetic with ET tube
B. General anaesthetic with iGel
C. Spinal anaesthetic with low dose bupivacaine
D. Epidural anaesthesia
E. No anaesthesia required

SBA 24:

An anaesthetic department wants to perform a survey to determine their anaesthetists' choice of opiate for major colorectal surgery. The department currently uses five different opiates and they wish to reduce their formulary down to two to become more cost-efficient.

Following the survey, what would be the most appropriate statistical test for analysing the data?

A. ANOVA
B. Student's unpaired t test
C. Regression analysis
D. Chi-squared test
E. Mann–Whitney U test

SBA 25:

A 26-year-old woman is 1 day post-partum. She is usually fit and well. She had a category 3 caesarean section for failure to progress, which was performed under spinal anaesthesia with no complications. The midwives are concerned as she is complaining of a band-like headache and would like a review.

What is the most likely cause of the patient's headache?

A. Post dural puncture headache
B. Cluster headache
C. Tension headache
D. Intracranial haemorrhage
E. Migraine

SBA 26:

A 71-year-old woman is undergoing an elective right hemi-colectomy for colon cancer. She has a history of rheumatoid arthritis, TMJ dysfunction, hypertension and gout. During induction of anaesthesia, she was haemodynamically stable, but had an unexpected difficult airway (requiring three attempts at laryngoscopy). The procedure continued smoothly, but following extubation she complains of some difficulty in moving her upper limbs bilaterally as well as sensory loss in her upper and lower body. There is less difficulty in moving the lower limbs.

What is the most likely diagnosis?

A. Central cord syndrome
B. Severe electrolyte imbalance
C. Cerebral infarction
D. Peripheral nerve injury
E. Spinal arteriovenous malformation

SBA 27:

A 62-year-old patient presents to A&E after having a fall. On reviewing the patient's past medical history, an echocardiogram performed this year indicates moderate aortic regurgitation.

What are the key haemodynamic goals peri-operatively?

A. Maintain blood pressure using vasopressors
B. Slow normal heart rate
C. Maximise preload
D. Prevent pulmonary vasoconstriction
E. Maintain forward flow of blood through the heart

SBA 28:

A previously fit and well 38-year-old man presents for hernia repair in day surgery. He undergoes general anaesthesia as well as having an ilioinguinal nerve block. Following the surgery he is complaining of leg weakness and is unable to mobilise.

What is the most likely cause of leg weakness?

A. Nerve palsy due to poor positioning intra-operatively
B. Inadvertent femoral nerve block
C. Surgical trauma to ilioinguinal nerve
D. Exacerbation of pre-existing sciatic nerve injury
E. Intraneural ilioinguinal nerve block

SBA 29:

With regard to the vascular network of the spinal cord, which of the following is incorrect?

A. Venous drainage is via 1 anterior and 2 posterior spinal veins
B. The anterior spinal artery is formed by branches of the vertebral arteries
C. The posterior spinal arteries originate from the vertebral artery
D. The largest anterior medullary artery is known as the artery of Adamkiewicz
E. The posterior spinal arteries anastomose with each other in the pia mater

SBA 30:

You are preparing a ventilated patient for repatriation to an intensive care unit closer to their family's home, requiring a 10-hour road transfer. The patient is on 50% oxygen and has a respiratory rate of 12 breaths per minute, with a tidal volume of 500ml. The ventilator requires 500ml of gas per minute as driving pressure.

What would be an appropriate number and size of cylinders to take on this journey? (The transport has only emergency piped supply)

A. 2 size E cylinders
B. 4 size E cylinders
C. 7 size E cylinders
D. 2 size F cylinders
E. 5 size F cylinders

SBA 31:

A 63-year-old patient has presented for a biopsy for a suspicious lesion on his right vocal cord. The ENT surgeons wish for high frequency jet ventilation to be used to improve surgical view and allow them to take a full and accurate biopsy.

With regard to the elimination of CO_2, which of the following parameters is the most important when changed in isolation?

A. Respiratory frequency
B. Inspiratory time
C. Driving pressure
D. Expiratory time
E. Peak airway pressure

SBA 32:

A 67-year-old patient is undergoing endovascular aneurysm repair (EVAR) for an abdominal aortic aneurysm. Following injection of contrast the radiologist describes the patient's aneurysm sac being filled by a branch of the inferior mesenteric artery.

What type of endoleak is the radiologist describing?

A. Type I endoleak
B. Type II endoleak
C. Type III endoleak
D. Type IV endoleak
E. Type V endoleak

SBA 33:

You review a 48-year-old woman in the chronic pain clinic, with a history of severe lower back pain. Her GP had referred her for a review due to worsening pain since increasing her morphine sulfate dose. She currently takes 1g paracetamol QDS, ibuprofen 400mg TDS, 120mg of a modified-release morphine preparation (MST) BD. She had been taking 80mg of modified-release MST BD prior to last week.

What is the most likely cause for the patient's increasing levels of pain?

A. Opioid dependence
B. Opioid addiction
C. Opioid tolerance
D. Opioid-induced hyperalgesia
E. Opioid-induced allodynia

SBA 34:

A 5-year-old boy is under anaesthesia for an inguinal hernia repair. The patient is taken into the operating theatre and upon exposing the child for surgery, you notice he is covered in bruises on the lower limb and abdomen.

What should be done next before the surgery commences?

A. Take photos of the bruises with medical photography for evidence
B. Continue with surgery and investigate further post-operatively
C. Pause surgery and ask the patient's parents about the bruising
D. Ask for a child safeguarding lead to attend theatre
E. Do not continue with surgery, wake the patient and discuss the bruises with the child and parents post-recovery

SBA 35:

A patient has been admitted to ICU for high flow nasal oxygen after developing type 1 respiratory failure on the respiratory ward. He has a diagnosis of active TB and is on combination therapy. He begins to complain of new onset blurred vision.

Which drug is the most likely cause of his visual disturbance?

A. Rifampicin
B. Isoniazid
C. Ethambutol
D. Pyrazinamide
E. Hydroxychloroquine

SBA 36:

Your colleague comes to discuss their case with you as they have inadvertently performed a wrong-sided block for a patient on their operating list.

The following are thought to increase risk of wrong-sided block except:

A. Mark or sticker placed by anaesthetic practitioner
B. >1 block performed
C. Patient repositioning
D. Use of mild sedation
E. Inadequate information from the patient

SBA 37:

A 26-year-old man has presented to the pre-assessment clinic with a familial history of malignant hyperthermia.

Which chromosome contains the responsible gene in susceptible individuals?

A. Chromosome 19
B. Chromosome 23
C. Chromosome 17
D. Chromosome 13
E. Chromosome 9

SBA 38:

A 28-year-old woman is 16 hours post-partum. She had an emergency caesarean section the previous evening due to sustained foetal bradycardia. She has been hypertensive throughout her pregnancy and was given a diagnosis of pre-eclampsia in clinic. She was placed on oral labetalol for blood pressure control. This has continued in the intra-partum and post-partum period. An arrest call is put out as the patient has started seizing.

What is the immediate pharmacological management of this patient?

A. IV lorazepam 4mg
B. PR diazepam 10mg
C. IV $MgSO_4$ 4g
D. IV phenytoin 1.5g
E. IV levetiracetam 750mg

SBA 39:

A 26-year-old patient presents to A&E with a reduced GCS. For 5 days prior to admission he was complaining of a headache and blurred vision. He vomited on arrival and has been intubated, ventilated and sedated. He had a CT scan which demonstrates a large enhancing lesion with midline shift. The neurosurgeons have been contacted, but are in theatre at the nearest neurosurgical centre which is 45 miles away.

What is the next pharmacological step in the patient's management?

A. Hypertonic saline 7ml/kg
B. IV acetazolamide 500mg
C. Mannitol 5g/kg
D. IV lorazepam 4mg
E. IV dexamethasone 6.6mg

SBA 40:

A 60-year-old patient has undergone successful mitral valve replacement on cardiopulmonary bypass. At the end of the operation, the patient's heart function is assessed via transoesophageal echo (TOE) prior to coming off cardiopulmonary bypass. The heart demonstrates a global lack of contractility and there is evidence of pulmonary hypertension.

What is the inotrope of choice in this scenario to facilitate weaning the patient off bypass?

A. Dobutamine
B. Milrinone
C. Levosimendan
D. Adrenaline
E. Dopexamine

SBA 41:

With regard to performing an ankle block on a patient for foot surgery, which nerve supplies the deep ventral structures and muscles of the foot?

A. Posterior tibial nerve
B. Sural nerve
C. Calcaneal nerve
D. Deep peroneal nerve
E. Superficial peroneal nerve

SBA 42:

The resting splanchnic blood flow is:

A. 20ml/min/100g of tissue
B. 30ml/min/100g of tissue
C. 40ml/min/100g of tissue
D. 50ml/min/100g of tissue
E. 60ml/min/100g of tissue

SBA 43:

A 48-year-old man is on the ENT ward having undergone a total thyroidectomy 18 hours ago. He has been becoming increasingly short of breath over the last 3 hours. On review by the ENT SHO he is found to be drooling and has a large expanding mass in the neck. He also has an audible stridor.

What is the immediate management of this patient?

A. Immediate scalpel cricothyroidotomy
B. Initiate high flow nasal oxygen
C. Transfer to theatre and prepare for emergency surgical tracheostomy
D. Immediate intubation and ventilation
E. Open strap muscles with surgical scissors

SBA 44:

You have anaesthetised a 62-year-old man for an elective suprarenal abdominal aorta repair.

Regarding the intra-operative conduct, which of the following is false regarding blood product/fluid management?

A. Aim to keep haemoglobin >90g/L
B. Aim to keep CVP >12–15mmHg
C. Aim to keep haemoglobin >70g/L
D. Crystalloid fluid loading can be used before aortic unclamping
E. Colloid fluid loading can be used before aortic unclamping

SBA 45:

Which of the following procedures is thought to be least painful for patients in ITU?

A. Removal of chest tubes
B. Wound care
C. Peripheral venepuncture
D. Arterial line insertion
E. Endotracheal tube suctioning

SBA 46:

A 25kg 8-year-old patient has presented for lipoma removal under general anaesthetic. He has a history of autism spectrum disorder, and after discussion with the child's parents in the pre-assessment clinic it had been agreed that the patient would require oral sedation prior to admission to the anaesthetic room.

What is the correct dose of oral midazolam for this patient?

A. 0.25mg
B. 6.25mg
C. 12.5mg
D. 25mg
E. 50mg

SBA 47:

An 18-year-old man is brought to the intensive care unit following an attempted suicide. It is unclear how long the patient was in cardiac arrest for, but the team in the resus department achieved return of spontaneous circulation (ROSC). He is transferred to the intensive care unit but after testing, is declared brainstem dead. His family have consented for organ donation. Overnight he becomes hypotensive despite multiple crystalloid boluses.

What is the next step in the patient's management?

A. Further IV fluid bolus of isotonic solution
B. Commence infusion of noradrenaline and titrate as required
C. Commence infusion of adrenaline and titrate as required
D. Commence infusion of phenylephrine and titrate as required
E. Commence infusion of vasopressin and titrate as required

SBA 48:

Which of the following risk factors is not associated with an increased risk of developing an inpatient venous thromboembolism (VTE)?

A. Hip or knee replacement
B. Chemotherapy
C. Varicose veins with phlebitis
D. Diabetes mellitus type 2
E. Age >50

CRQs and SBAs for the Final FRCA

SBA 49:

A 58-year-old patient on the ITU has been proned following periods of difficult gas exchange secondary to acute respiratory distress syndrome. He is being mechanically ventilated through an endotracheal tube.

Which of the following statements most accurately represents the distribution of ventilation in this patient?

A. Predominantly in the dependent lung (dorsal)
B. Uniform ventilation across entire lung
C. Predominantly in the non-dependent lung (ventral)
D. Predominantly in the non-dependent lung (dorsal)
E. Predominantly in the dependent lung (ventral)

SBA 50:

Which of the following is suggestive of a 'non-reassuring' foetal cardiotocography trace?

A. Baseline at 140bpm, variability 10bpm, variable decelerations with no concerning characteristics for 10 minutes
B. Baseline at 110bpm, variability 20bpm, variable decelerations with no concerning characteristics for 60 minutes
C. Baseline at 160bpm, variability 30bpm, variable decelerations with no concerning characteristics for 90 minutes
D. Baseline at 150bpm, variability 25bpm, variable decelerations with no concerning characteristics for 80 minutes
E. Baseline at 110bpm, variability 5bpm, variable decelerations with no concerning characteristics for 5 minutes

SBA 51:

A 38-year-old woman presents to A&E with a progressive shortness of breath and expiratory stridor.

What is the first-line investigation to determine the cause of her stridor?

A. CT head and neck
B. Chest X-ray
C. Nasendoscopy
D. MRI neck
E. Full blood count

SBA 52:

A 71-year-old woman is due to undergo cataract surgery. You have discussed a sub-Tenon's block with the patient, who has no contraindications to this approach.

What is the most appropriate method to prepare the patient's eye for the sub-Tenon's block?

A. 0.5% proxymetacaine eye drops
B. 2% tetracaine eye drops
C. 3% lidocaine eye peribulbar injection
D. 0.25% levobupivacaine peri-orbital injection
E. 1% lidocaine eye drops

SBA 53:

Which medication is not recommended by NICE for first-line management of acute pain crisis in sickle cell disease?

A. Paracetamol
B. NSAIDs
C. Pethidine
D. Weak opioids
E. Strong opioids IV

SBA 54:

A 5-year-old boy is listed for an elective insertion of grommets under general anaesthesia. In the pre-operative waiting area, he has EMLA (eutectic mixture of local anaesthetic) cream applied to facilitate cannulation and oral midazolam to alleviate anxiety. In the anaesthetic room, he has an uneventful induction and an LMA is inserted. The ODP notices the patient has become cyanotic despite 100% oxygen. An ABG is taken which shows a PaO_2 of 40kPa.

What is the first-line treatment for this patient?

A. Prostaglandin infusion
B. Exchange transfusion
C. Methylene blue
D. Hyperbaric oxygen therapy
E. Riboflavin

SBA 55:

A 58-year-old man presented to hospital with shortness of breath and a productive cough. He is diagnosed with chest sepsis, and transferred to the intensive care unit. He has been given 3L of fluid on the ward but remains hypotensive and tachycardic. The patient is intubated and ventilated, and has a central line *in situ*. Cardiac output monitoring is commenced via a pulmonary artery catheter, and the following variables are calculated:

GEDI (global end-diastolic index) – 500ml/m^2
SVV (stroke volume variation) – 11%
SVRI (systemic vascular resistance index) – 2000/dyn/sec/cm^{-5}/m^2
EVLWI (extravascular lung water index) – 5ml/kg

What is the next step in the patient's management?

A. Further IV fluid bolus of isotonic solution
B. Commence infusion of noradrenaline and titrate as required
C. No changes to current management
D. Commence infusion of dobutamine and titrate as required
E. Increase speed of propofol infusion

SBA 56:

A 65-year-old man scheduled for an elective cholecystectomy is reviewed in the pre-operative assessment clinic. He has a background of chronic obstructive pulmonary disease (COPD) and smokes approximately 20 cigarettes per day.

Which of the following is not true regarding smoking?

A. Smoking causes a reduction in FEV_1
B. Smoking is an inducer of CYP2E1 activity
C. The half-life of nicotine is 30 minutes
D. Smoking causes a rightward shift in the oxygen haemoglobin dissociation curve
E. There is a dose-dependent relationship between smoking and subarachnoid haemorrhage

SBA 57:

A patient has been anaesthetised for an elective laparoscopic hysterectomy. The patient was given an intubating dose of rocuronium at the start of the operation. At the end of the operation a 'train-of-four' is used via the nerve stimulator to check the level of neuromuscular blockade and reversibility. There are three twitches present.

What does this correspond to in terms of receptor occupancy by the neuromuscular blocking agent?

A. 80%
B. 75%
C. 65%
D. 40%
E. 30%

SBA 58:

With regard to regional and neuraxial anaesthesia, which site of injection has the greatest absorption and therefore propensity to develop local anaesthetic toxicity?

A. Interscalene
B. Supraclavicular
C. Intercostal
D. Epidural
E. Spinal

SBA 59:

A patient is undergoing cardiopulmonary bypass for a coronary artery bypass grafting (CABG). The surgeons are ready to insert the bypass catheters but wish for the patient to be appropriately anticoagulated.

What is the target activated clotting time (ACT) in seconds to insert aortic and vena cava catheters after administration of IV heparin?

A. 400s
B. 440s
C. 480s
D. 520s
E. 560s

SBA 60:

A 45-year-old female patient has been transferred to the post-operative high dependency unit following trans-sphenoidal surgery for a pituitary adenoma. 7 hours post-operatively she is passing large volumes of dilute urine and has a sodium of 155mmol/L on a venous blood gas.

What is the most likely cause?

A. Diabetes insipidus
B. Excess IV fluid intra-operatively
C. Addisonian crisis
D. Stress response to surgery
E. SIADH

CRQ 1: answer guidance

Syllabus	NU_IK_06, PR_IK_04
Question type	Hard: pass mark 10
Topic	**Pharmacokinetics of sepsis**
Aim	To understand the changes in pharmacokinetics and drug handling that severe sepsis has on patients, specifically those in the ICU setting.
Pass requirements	The correct definition of sepsis and its underlying pathology.

Q	Answer	Marks	Guidance
a	• An overwhelming and life-threatening response to infection • that can cause tissue damage, organ failure and ultimately death if left untreated	1 1	This is the most recent definition as per the UK Sepsis Trust, and although it has had many iterations, the principles are the same.
b	• Widespread release of cytokines and reactive oxygen species, leading to direct or indirect cellular damage • Vasodilation and capillary leak occur, leading to absolute intravascular hypovolaemia • Impaired microcirculatory blood flow leading to impaired perfusion, mitochondrial dysfunction and ultimately cellular hypoxia	1 1 1	The sequence of events leading to cell damage should be straightforward. The wording does not have to be identical, but key concepts such as vasodilation or mitochondrial dysfunction should not be excluded.
c	**Absorption:** • Delayed gastric emptying in critically unwell or ileus if post-operative • Decreased splanchnic blood flow due to vasopressive agents • Use of opiates for sedation may slow gastric transit • Mucosal oedema • Suctioning NG tubes regularly • Alterations of intraluminal pH • Reduced skin or muscle perfusion from redistributed blood flow	4	1 mark per correct answer (maximum marks for each part detailed in column). Drug pharmacokinetics can be changed significantly during sepsis. Primarily, this is driven by changes in the volume of distribution, and alterations of liver and kidney function. It is important to have an understanding of these changes as many drugs may reach toxic levels at previously normal dosages, leading to long-term morbidity. An example of this would be gentamicin.

Q	Answer	Marks	Guidance
	Distribution: • Changes in volume of distribution (increased Vd in hydrophilic medications due to capillary leak and fluid shift or redistribution from peripheral tissues) • Changes in pKa will influence movement across capillary membranes – acidaemia is frequently encountered in sepsis • Changes in protein levels (albumin and alpha1 glycoprotein) can alter drug binding and therefore Vd	3	
	Metabolism: • Abnormalities in hepatic function may alter degree of metabolism of hepatic drugs (reduction in hepatic perfusion or changes in cytochrome p450 dynamics)	1	
	Elimination: • Abnormalities in renal function can change elimination of drugs, specifically those that undergo renal excretion. This may be due to AKI, changes in renal perfusion or alteration of elimination dynamics if the patient is on renal replacement therapy.	1	
d	• Propofol is highly lipid-soluble, with extensive protein binding in normal physiology • Initially volume of distribution is decreased due to a centralisation of blood flow • There is a decrease in serum albumin • This can lead to higher free plasma concentrations, and exaggerate cardiovascular side-effects • Decreased cardiac output then delays the effects from changes to dose; e.g. induction of sedation may take longer • Renal or hepatic dysfunction have limited effects on propofol metabolism, as it has inactive metabolites • Prolonged infusion leads to increased context-sensitive half-life	3	1 mark per correct answer. Propofol is the most common anaesthetic drug used in daily practice, and in critical care it is often used for sedation. It is useful to know that small changes in dose can give large changes in cardiovascular output, as this exaggerated response can have severe consequences.

Q	Answer	Marks	Guidance
e	• Tachyphylaxis does occur with increasing duration of use • Down-regulation of catecholamine receptors • Increased nitric oxide and prostacyclin production • Further generation of oxygen free radicals • Activation of ATP-sensitive potassium channels (via prolonged acidaemia) which causes hyper-polarisation and vasodilation	3	1 mark per correct answer. 1 mark can be given here for identifying the pharmacokinetic principle of tachyphylaxis. This concept is why vasopressors such as vasopressin are added alongside noradrenaline in severe sepsis. Because of their short half-life, pharmacokinetic variability is usually not an issue in critical care.

Altered pharmacokinetics in the context of sepsis is frequently encountered in both anaesthetic practice and critical care. The understanding of pharmacokinetics is encountered in the primary FRCA exam; however, the ability to contextualise and understand the relevance is important in clinical practice and the final FRCA curriculum. The precise effect of sepsis on pharmacokinetics is hard to predict due to the variable host response. Absorption has the most variability. Care should be taken when using vasoactive drugs but specifically those with a narrow therapeutic range as they can quickly develop toxic levels and toxic effects.

Charlton, M. and Thompson, J. (2019) Pharmacokinetics in sepsis. *BJA Education*, **19(1):** 7–13.

Rudd, K., Johnson, S., Agesa, K. *et al.* (2020) Global, regional, and national sepsis incidence and mortality, 1990-2017: analysis for the Global Burden of Disease Study. *Lancet*, **395(10219):** 200–11.

CRQ 2: answer guidance

Syllabus	OB_IK_09, VS_IK_12
Question type	Easy: pass mark 13
Topic	**Major obstetric haemorrhage and intra-operative blood product management**
Aim	To understand the management of the major obstetric patient as well as the peri-operative management of the patient at high risk of bleeding but refusing blood products
Pass requirements	Ability to label and understand the TEG trace and appreciate its use in haemorrhage

Q	Answer	Marks	Guidance
a	• Haemodilution – physiological anaemia due to increase in blood volume • Reduction in number of platelets • Absolute reduction in red cell number • Prothrombotic state due to venous stasis and increase in clotting factors	3	1 mark per correct answer. Reduction in number of platelets can be variable between patients but there is still a reduction in number. Prothrombotic state puts these patients at high risk of developing DVT and PE.
b	**Pre-op:** • IV iron therapy • Injection of erythropoietin • Pre-op autologous blood donation (if acceptable to patient) **Intra-op:** • Cell salvage • Use of other blood products (e.g. cryoprecipitate) • Intra-op cell salvage • Tranexamic acid injection/infusion	2 2	2 marks each for pre-op and post-op. Depending on the patient, they may be amenable to blood transfusion so this would need to be elucidated in pre-assessment clinic.
c	**Advantages:** • Avoid risk of autologous blood transfusion • May be more acceptable to the patient • Avoids use of hospital blood stores • Cheaper than use of cross-matched blood **Disadvantages:** • Need for specific training • Theoretical risk of amniotic fluid embolus • No clotting factors contained	3 3	3 marks each for disadvantages and advantages.
d	• Lack of trained staff available • Complete patient refusal	1	These are the most recent contraindications. AFE considered theoretical.

Q	Answer	Marks	Guidance
e	**1** R time/activation time/clotting time: time from start of test to initial fibrin formation (depends on clotting factors) **2** K time/clot formation time: time to achieve certain clot strength – amplitude of 20mm (depends on fibrinogen) **3** Alpha angle: speed of fibrin build-up and cross-linking takes place (depends on fibrinogen) **4** Maximum clot firmness: the ultimate strength/stability of the clot **5** LY30/clot lysis time: decrease in the maximum amplitude	5	1 mark per correct answer. It is not necessary to include which clotting factors/processes each of these corresponds with.
f	• Hypercoagulable state with secondary fibrinolysis • Decreased R and K time, increased alpha angle and maximum amplitude • Smaller lysis 30	1	Classically the trace will be bell-shaped (wider, and with a shorter lead time). The smaller lysis 30 corresponds to early clot breakdown.

Blood loss is common in obstetric surgery; however, most patients are amenable to blood transfusion. There are a subset of patients who refuse blood transfusions, and these are not restricted to Jehovah's Witnesses. Any patient who would refuse blood transfusion should be seen in anaesthetic pre-assessment clinic to discuss their options and to understand what a patient may accept. TEG or ROTEM is a useful point of care test if there is an obstetric haemorrhage, as it allows for specific blood product replacement. It is especially useful if the patient will accept derived blood products, but not blood itself. Previous fears of amniotic fluid embolism in the use of intra-operative cell salvage have not been proven, and there is no concrete evidence to restrict its use.

Carroll, C. and Young, F. (2021) Intra-operative cell salvage. *BJA Education*, **21(3):** 95–101.

Plaat, F. and Shonfield, A. (2015) Major obstetric haemorrhage. *BJA Education*, **15(4):** 190–193.

CRQ 3: answer guidance

Syllabus	MT_IK_02, MT_IK_04, PB_IK_28
Question type	Moderate: pass mark 13
Topic	**Management of traumatic brain injury**
Aim	To be able to correctly describe the initial management of the patient who has sustained a head injury.
Pass requirements	Show understanding of strategies to reduce secondary traumatic brain injury.

Q	Answer	Marks	Guidance
a	• Coma • Significantly decreasing conscious level (<2 GCS in an hour) • Loss of laryngeal reflexes • Insufficient ventilation • Spontaneous hyperventilation • Irregular respiratory pattern/rate • Copious bleeding into mouth • Seizures	6	1 mark per correct answer. Accept GCS <8, i.e. decrease in GCS motor score by 1 or more points. i.e. pO_2 <13kPa or pCO_2 >6kPa. i.e. spontaneous respiration to pCO_2 <4kPa. Accept unstable facial fractures or bilateral mandible fractures.
b	• GCS <15 on initial assessment • Neck pain or focal tenderness • Focal neurological deficit • Paraesthesia in extremities • Clinical suspicion of cervical spine injury	4	1 mark per correct answer.
c	**Advantage:** • Reduced risk of cardiovascular instability **Disadvantages:** • Unfamiliarity with use • Does not act within 1 arm–brain circulation time • May increase MAP and therefore ICP	1 1	The rise in MAP (and ICP) is controversial, with most guidance showing that the rise in MAP is negligible.
d	• Further injury to the brain as a result of the initial injury mediated by inflammatory and neurotoxic processes • Timeframe: hours to days	1 1	Can accept a specific number for timeframe. The key point is that it occurs later than the primary brain injury.
e	• 60–70mmHg	1	
f	• Mannitol 0.25–1g/kg • Hypertonic saline 2ml/kg • Normoxia • Hyperventilation • Controlled hypothermia • Barbiturate coma • Decompressive craniectomy • Extraventricular drain insertion	5	1 mark per correct answer. Can accept hyperventilation expressed in $paCO_2$ 4–4.5kPa as well as normoxia with PaO_2 >13kPa.

Head injuries can present in any hospital, typically as a trauma call. As a result, anaesthetists are expected to have a thorough knowledge of the management of a head injury patient. There are easily available NICE guidelines on the management strategies for these patients, until such time that they can be transferred to either a neurosurgical unit for definitive management, or a neuro-intensive care unit for further observation.

Brain Trauma Foundation (2016) *Guidelines for the Management of Severe TBI*, 4th ed.

Dinsmore, J. (2013) Traumatic brain injury: an evidence-based review of management. *CEACCP*, **13(6)**: 189–195.

NICE (2014; updated 2019) *Head Injury: assessment and early management* [CG176].

CRQ 4: answer guidance

Syllabus	AM_IK_01, AM_IS_01
Question type	Easy: pass mark 14
Topic	**Awake fibre-optic intubation**
Aim	To be able to confidently describe the anatomy relating to an awake fibre-optic intubation and the complications that can be associated with its placement.
Pass requirements	Correctly identify the complications of an AFOI.

Q	Answer	Marks	Guidance
a	**Indications:** • Known or predicted difficult airway • High risk of aspiration • Inability to access pre-tracheal or cricoid region • Cervical spine instability needing in-line stabilisation **Contraindications:** • Patient refusal • Allergy to local anaesthetic agents • Blood in airway • Coagulopathy (if using nasal route) • Peri-glottic masses or stridulous patients	3	1 mark per 2 correct answers. Base of skull fracture may also be a relative contraindication; however, in fibre-optic intubation direct visualisation throughout should avoid any damage through the fracture. The absolute contraindications are refusal or allergy; others are relative. No half marks so 1 mark per pair.
b	**Nose:** anterior ethmoidal nerve (from ophthalmic nerve), greater palatine nerve, lesser palatine nerve (from maxillary nerve) **Pharynx:** glossopharyngeal nerve **Oropharynx:** tonsillar nerve (from glossopharyngeal nerve), lingual nerve (from vagus) **Larynx:** internal branch of the superior laryngeal nerve (above cords), recurrent laryngeal (below cords) – both are branches of the vagus nerve	6	1 mark per correct answer. These are all terminal branches that supply the airway tract for awake fibre-optic. Candidates should be confident in naming 6 of these nerves.
c	9ml/kg lidocaine	1	
d	2.5ml of co-phenylcaine contains 125mg of lidocaine and 12.5mg of phenylcaine	1	Co-phenylcaine is recommended for airway topicalisation in the DAS guidelines as a local analgesic, and as a vasoconstrictor.

Q	Answer	Marks	Guidance
e	• Remifentanil Minto TCI (Ce 1–3ng/ml) • Midazolam 0.5–1mg if second anaesthetist present • Propofol (TCI only – not bolus) • Dexmedetomidine	2	1 mark per correct answer. Doses are not necessary but if listing midazolam, it is important to note that there must be a second anaesthetist present.
f	• Capnography trace • Auscultation of breath sounds • Misting of the ETT/angle piece • Direct visualisation with fibre-optic scope • Direct visualisation with standard or video laryngoscope	2	1 mark per correct answer. DAS recommends the use of a 2-point check which includes capnography.
g	**Over-sedation:** vomiting and aspiration, obtunded airway reflexes, loss of airway **Topicalisation:** local anaesthetic toxicity, anaphylaxis, pain **Hypoxia:** hypoventilation, hypoxia **Performance:** failure, bleeding, airway swelling, perforation of cuff, oesophageal intubation, mucous/secretion plugging	5	1 mark for each. The complications can be split into the 4 main headings for ease of categorisation.

Awake fibre-optic intubation should be in the back pocket for every anaesthetist who comes up against a predicted difficult airway. Recent guidelines (2020) have been issued by the Difficult Airway Society to make the technique more uniform, as prior to this there were (and still are) multiple ways in which to perform it. It is essential to have an understanding of the underlying anatomy, as this question is asked regularly in Royal College exams.

Ahmad, I., El-Boghdadly, K., Bhagrath, R. *et al.* (2020) Difficult Airway Society guidelines for awake tracheal intubation (ATI) in adults. *Anaesthesia*, **75(4):** 509–528.

Leslie, D. and Stacey, M. (2015) Awake intubation. *BJA Education*, **15(2):** 64–67.

CRQ 5: answer guidance

Syllabus	NA_IK_12, PM_IK_06, PM_IS_03
Question type	Easy: pass mark 14
Topic	**Trigeminal neuralgia**
Aim	To recall the anatomy relevant to trigeminal neuralgia, the diagnostic criteria and pharmacotherapy.
Pass requirements	Demonstrate an understanding of the trigeminal nerve anatomy and trigeminal neuralgia.

Q	Answer	Marks	Guidance
a	• Multiple sclerosis • Increasing age • Previous stroke • Hypertension • Charcot–Marie–Tooth disease • Trigeminal nerve root tumours • Trauma	5	1 mark per correct answer. Can also accept space-occupying lesion in place of trigeminal nerve root tumours.
b	• V1 – superior orbital fissure • V2 – foramen rotundum • V3 – foramen ovale	1 1 1	
c	• Paroxysmal attacks lasting seconds • In the division of the trigeminal nerve • Pain described as sharp/stabbing/intense or superficial • Attacks stereotyped in the individual patient • No neurological deficit • Not caused by another disorder	3	1 mark per correct answer. Accept attack lasting <2 mins. Can include one of the pain descriptors only.
d	• Carbamazepine – anticonvulsant – sodium channel (use-dependent) • Gabapentin – anticonvulsant – (voltage-gated) calcium channel • Amitriptyline – tricyclic antidepressant – voltage-gated Na^+ channels, voltage-gated K^+ channels, alpha1 adrenergic receptor, alpha2 adrenergic receptor, dopamine receptor, histamine receptor, muscarinic acetylcholine receptor, serotonin receptor, noradrenaline receptor, dopamine receptor (1 of)	1 + 1 1 + 1 1 + 1	

Q	Answer	Marks	Guidance
e	• Peripheral lysis of trigeminal nerve branches • Gasserian ganglion ablation • Microvascular decompression • Gamma knife stereotactic radio-surgery	3	1 mark per correct answer. Can accept laser or ETOH lysis of nerve. Can accept radiofrequency/chemical/mechanical ablation of ganglion.

Whilst trigeminal neuralgia has very defined symptoms and signs, its treatment is often difficult. Diagnosis can be challenging due to the overlap with other syndromes. Management is either medical or surgical, but surgical treatment is often major neurosurgery and is avoided as much as possible. Nevertheless, the condition can be debilitating and comes with significant morbidity.

Vasappa, C., Kapur, S. and Krovvidi, H. (2016) Trigeminal neuralgia. *BJA Education*, **16(10):** 353–356.

Yao, A. and Barad, M. (2020) Diagnosis and management of chronic facial pain. *BJA Education*, **20(4):** 120–125.

CRQ 6: answer guidance

Syllabus	PA_IK_02
Question type	Hard: pass mark 10
Topic	**Congenital diaphragmatic hernia**
Aim	To be able to recognise CDH, instigate initial management and understand when a patient is fit for corrective surgery.
Pass requirements	Recall which patients have a likely poor outcome.

Q	Answer	Marks	Guidance
a	• Respiratory distress • Scaphoid abdomen	1 1	A scaphoid abdomen is a sunken anterior abdominal wall.
b	• Abdominal organs within the thoracic cavity	1	
c	• Trisomy 13 • Trisomy 18 • Trisomy 21 • Fryns syndrome • Cornelia de Lange syndrome • CHARGE syndrome	2	1 mark per correct answer. Structural abnormalities are not listed here, as this is about genetics.
d	• Ventricular septal defect • Atrial septal defect • Coarctation of the aorta • Hypoplastic left heart	2	1 mark per correct answer. Others do exist but are much rarer.

Q	Answer	Marks	Guidance
e	• Large defect size • Associated cardiac abnormalities • Associated chromosomal abnormalities • Severe pulmonary hypertension • Low birth weight • Low APGAR score at 5 mins • Small contralateral lung • Bilateral CHD	4	1 mark per correct answer. Each of these contribute to poor outcome. Other concurrent illness such as post-delivery sepsis could also gain 1 mark.
f	• *Initial resus* including IV access and fluid therapy • *Early intubation and ventilation* to prevent respiratory distress • *Insertion of NG tube* to decompress bowel • *Echocardiogram*	3	1 mark per correct answer. The mainstays of management should be resuscitation and gaining control of ventilation in those with respiratory distress. Echocardiogram is essential as it quantifies degree of pulmonary HTN, cardiac defects or conduction abnormalities and is used to guide further management.
g	• **Prostaglandins:** helps offload right side of the heart by maintaining ductus patency • **Inotropes/vasopressors:** to maintain blood pressure in the critically unwell • **Neuromuscular blockers:** can improve chest wall compliance if the patient is ventilated • **Sildenafil/prostacyclin** to treat refractory pulmonary hypertension	3	1 mark per correct answer. Can accept specific drug names. NB: nitric oxide has not been shown to improve outcome and is associated with increased mortality so should not be used.
h	• MAP normal for gestation • Lactate <3mmol/L • Urine output >1ml/kg/hr • Preductal O_2 sats 85–95% on FiO_2 <0.5	3	1 mark per correct answer. It is important to note that if the patient is already on ECMO this does not apply.

This is a challenging question for a variety of reasons. 50% or more of CDHs are now diagnosed *in utero* and techniques to operate on those whilst *in utero* are becoming more common. However, many can be missed, and although a rare presentation, it is not beyond the realms of possibility that one could be faced with this out of hours in a small hospital. The management is complex and will often need two consultant paediatric anaesthetists as a minimum; however, knowing the fundamentals underpinning the pathology is of some use in the acute management.

Quinney, M. and Wellesley, H. (2018) Anaesthetic management of patients with a congenital diaphragmatic hernia. *BJA Education*, **18(4):** 95–101.

Snoek, K., Reiss, I., Greenough, A. *et al.* (2016) Standardized postnatal management of infants with congenital diaphragmatic hernia in Europe: the CDH EURO consortium consensus 2015 update. *Neonatology*, **110:** 66e74.

CRQ 7: answer guidance

Syllabus	OR_IK_01, OR_IS_01
Question type	Moderate: pass mark 13
Topic	**Bone cement implantation syndrome (BCIS)**
Aim	To describe bone cement implantation syndrome, its aetiology and surgical methods for its prevention.
Pass requirements	Knowledge of the underlying risk factors for development of bone cement implantation syndrome.

Q	Answer	Marks	Guidance
a	• Polymethyl methacrylate (PMMA)	1	Bone cement mainly contains PMMA but can also contain radio-opaque material and antibiotics. It also contains a liquid monomer (MMA).
b	• Can be used to provide strength to a joint which already contains osteoporosis • Antibiotics can be added to the cement • Cement can be quick drying so the operating surgeon can be confident the joint is stable quickly • Increases longevity of the joint in question	2	1 mark per correct answer. There is also a slight cost benefit to the use of a cemented joint likely to be due to longevity, therefore this cannot be considered a separate mark.
c	• Gentamicin • Vancomycin • Cefuroxime • Tobramycin	2	1 mark per correct answer. These are the most commonly used antibiotics in bone cement, so they should be avoided in patients with a documented allergy to them.
d	• The mechanical structure of the cement can be altered by the addition of antibiotics, making it weaker • Systemic toxicity • Increased cost to manufacture • Allergy and anaphylaxis • Renal failure precipitated by aminoglycosides • Antibiotic resistance	3	1 mark per correct answer. The mechanical structure issue is overcome by using less than 1g per 40g of antibiotics. More than 1g has physical implications.

Q	Answer	Marks	Guidance
e	**Patient factors:** ASA3/4, pre-existing pulmonary hypertension, significant cardiac disease, osteoporosis	2	1 mark per correct answer. Patients with any of these factors should be offered an un-cemented arthroplasty.
	Surgical factors: Pathological fractures, intertrochanteric fractures, long stem arthroplasty	2	
f	**Grade I:** moderate hypoxia (<94%) or a decrease in systolic BP by >20% **Grade II:** severe hypoxia (sats <88%), decrease in systolic blood pressure by >40%, or unexpected loss of consciousness **Grade III:** cardiovascular collapse	3	1 mark for each correct grade. Note how in each of these grades only one sign needs to change by the designated amount to increase the grade of the BCIS. This grading is from a 2009 article in the *BJA* and has not been updated since.
g	**Monomer model:** Circulating MMA monomers cause direct vasodilation	1	The monomer model has only ever been shown *in vitro* and not *in vivo* models due to the low circulating concentration of monomers.
	Embolus model: Marrow, fat, cement molecules and air can release inflammatory mediators and severely increase pulmonary vascular resistance, leading to cardiovascular collapse	1	No half marks so one mark per description. Can accept parts of description.
h	• Lavage of intramedullary canal • Good haemostasis prior to cementing • Drilling a venting hole in bone shaft • Retrograde insertion of cement • Use of vacuum within a proximal drainage cannula to reduce embolic load	3	1 mark per correct answer. Whilst there are no robust anaesthetic prevention techniques, it is still essential to understand what can be achieved surgically. The primary way to avoid BCIS would be to use an uncemented prosthesis.

Bone cement implantation syndrome is still poorly understood, but is a significant cause of both mortality and morbidity in the population undergoing hemi-arthroplasty. There are over 60 000 hip replacements in the NHS each year, and many of these patients will have risk factors for developing BCIS. Most of the time this will be grade I BCIS, and will not have any significant clinical consequence – but it can rapidly proceed to grade III. Anaesthetically, the best way to avoid BCIS is rigorous patient selection and pre-optimisation prior to surgery. High risk patients should have intra-operative cardiac output monitoring, and early use of vasopressors and fluid loading prior to cementing could be considered.

Donaldson, A., Thomson, H., Harper, N. and Kenny, N. (2009) Bone cement implantation syndrome. *BJA*, **102(1):** 12–22.

Khanna, G. and Cernovsky, J. (2012) Bone cement and the implications for anaesthesia. *CEACCP*, **12(4):** 213–216.

CRQ 8: answer guidance

Syllabus	TF_IK_09, MT_IK_05
Question type	Moderate: pass mark 13
Topic	**Burns management in adults**
Aim	To calculate the initial fluid resuscitation target in burns patients, as well as when to refer to a regional burns centre.
Pass requirements	Identify the possible indications for airway management in burns patients.

Q	Answer	Marks	Guidance
a	• Patient body surface area: 54% • 4ml × 36% × 90kg • 12960ml • 6480ml in first 8 hours, 6480ml in next 16 hours	1 1 1 1	The chest is 18% and each arm is 9% as per the Parkland formula, so the total BSA is 36%.
b	• Stridor • Hypoxaemia • Hypercarbia • GCS <8 • Deep facial burns • Full thickness neck burns • Oropharyngeal oedema	5	1 mark per correct answer. Each of these should prompt early airway assessment and possible management. It is better to intubate patients early with any of these signs, to prevent a difficult airway later on when there is possible oedema.
c	• Tube should be uncut • Tube should be 8.0 or above • Video-laryngoscopy is advised in case of early laryngeal swelling • Suxamethonium should be avoided if fire started >24 hours ago • There may be other trauma obscured by low GCS so may need C-spine immobilisation • Risk of cardiac arrest due to hypovolaemia at induction	3	1 mark per correct answer. Each of these are possible considerations. Could also accept failure to secure airway, although this is a much more non-specific consideration.
d	• All burns >3% BSA in adults (2% in children) • All full thickness burns • All circumferential burns • Any burn with suspicion of non-accidental injury (for expert opinion) • All burns to hands, feet, face, perineum or genitals • Any chemical/electrical/friction burn • Any cold injury (cold burn) • Any unwell febrile child with burn	5	1 mark per correct answer. This is as per the national burn care referral guidance, produced by the National Network for Burn Care.

continued overleaf

Q	Answer	Marks	Guidance
	• Any concern regarding additional injuries that may prevent burn healing • Any signs of infection • Any suspicion of toxic shock syndrome • Intubated patients with burns		
e	• Deep vein thrombosis • Stress ulcers • ARDS/pulmonary oedema • Renal failure • Hypothermia • Infection of burn or other body system • Compartment syndrome	3	1 mark per correct answer. Infection should only be accepted once, and should also include the overarching diagnosis of sepsis (i.e. cannot award 2 marks for urine/chest infection). Later complications might include PTSD and pulmonary fibrosis.

Burns can present to any hospital at any time, and should be considered as a trauma. Key principles in burns management include early fluid resuscitation and airway management if necessary. The patient may need early surgical management and debridement, and should be assessed for this immediately. This may include discussion with the regional burns centre or on-call burns consultant; possibly also the on-call major trauma consultant. Do not forget that these patients may be intrinsic trauma patients so may need C-spine immobilisation and/or other trauma management which may complicate resuscitation. When considering airway management always use an uncut tube, as the tube may migrate secondary to laryngeal swelling.

Bishop, S. and Maguire, S. (2012) Anaesthesia and intensive care for major burns. *CEACCP*, **12(3):** 118–122.

National Network for Burn Care (2012) *National Burn Care Referral Guidance*. Available from: www.britishburnassociation.org/wp-content/uploads/2018/02/National-Burn-Care-Referral-Guidance-2012.pdf (accessed 19 January 2022).

Suman, A. and Owen, J. (2020) Update on the management of burns in paediatrics. *BJA Education*, **20(3):** 103–110.

CRQ 9: answer guidance

Syllabus	CT_IK_14, CT_IS_03
Question type	Hard: pass mark 13
Topic	**Intra-aortic balloon pump**
Aim	To understand the indications, contraindications and physiological outcomes of an IABP as well as strategies for weaning.
Pass requirements	The indications for the insertion of an IABP.

Q	Answer	Marks	Guidance
a	• To improve the ventricular performance of the failing heart • This is achieved by increasing myocardial oxygen delivery; • and reducing myocardial oxygen demand	2	The intra-aortic balloon pump reduces afterload, and therefore reduces myocardial oxygen demand. Oxygen delivery (via improved blood flow through the coronary arteries) improves during diastole. 1 mark for each of the correct statements.
b	• Acute myocardial infarction • Cardiogenic shock • Acute MR and VSD • During catheterisation and angioplasty • Refractory unstable angina • Weaning from cardiopulmonary bypass • Refractory LV failure • Refractory LV arrhythmia • Cardiomyopathy • Sepsis • Complex cardiac abnormalities in children	2	There are a number of indications for the insertion of an IABP. Most of these prevent worsening of the underlying pathology. No half marks, so 1 mark per correct pair.
c	• Aortic regurgitation • Aortic dissection • Chronic end-stage heart disease with no suggestion of recovery • Aortic stents	3	1 mark per correct answer. These are all absolute contraindications. Relative contraindications include uncontrolled sepsis, AAA, tachyarrhythmia, severe peripheral vascular disease.
d	**Aorta:** reduced systolic pressure, increased diastolic pressure **Left ventricle:** reduced systolic pressure, reduced end-diastolic pressure, reduced volume, reduced wall tension **Heart:** reduced afterload, reduced preload, increased cardiac output **Blood flow:** increased or unchanged coronary blood flow	4	1 mark for each correct anatomical area. These are the key haemodynamic effects at each area, with the overall effect being as described in **a**.
e	Helium: low density, so facilitates rapid transfer of gas from console to balloon	2	Helium is also rapidly absorbed into the bloodstream, making it a safer alternative to other gases such as nitrogen.

Q	Answer	Marks	Guidance
f	**1** Unassisted aortic end-diastolic pressure **2** Non-augmented systolic pressure **3** Augmented diastolic pressure **4** Reduced aortic end-diastolic pressure	4	1 mark per correct answer. This is an arterial waveform taken when IABP is *in situ*. The augmented pressures are what is important here, as this will improve coronary flow and also reduce afterload.
g	CPP = ADP – LVEDP	1	Coronary perfusion pressure is the difference between the aortic diastolic pressure and the left ventricular end-diastolic pressure.
h	• Can start when inotropic requirements are minimal • Reduce rate of augmented beats gradually from 1:1 to 1:2 then 1:3 • Can decrease the balloon volume systematically	2	1 mark per correct answer. Caution: the balloon should never be turned off *in situ* if patient is not anticoagulated, because of the risk of thrombus on the balloon.

Intra-aortic balloon pumping is the most widely used circulatory assist device for patients with severe cardiac failure. Despite this, its use in recent years has declined due to perceived complications. It is still not uncommon to see in clinical practice, especially after cardiac surgery, and so anaesthetists should be confident with being able to monitor for complications and troubleshoot. Complications to look out for include compartment syndrome, renal failure, haemolysis and air embolism. Weaning from an IABP can be done gradually in ICU or CCU, and patients can be awake while it is in use.

Krishna, M. and Zacharowski, K. (2009) Principles of intra-aortic balloon pump counter-pulsation. *CEACCP*, **9(1):** 24–28.

CRQ 10: answer guidance

Syllabus	POM_IS_22, PC_IK_22
Question type	Easy: pass mark 14
Topic	**Accidental awareness under anaesthesia**
Aim	To be able to define awareness and appreciate the different types.
Pass requirements	List the risk factors for the development of awareness under anaesthesia.

Q	Answer	Marks	Guidance
a	**Explicit memory/awareness:** Events can be consciously recalled, either spontaneously or on questioning; may include recall of events, conversations, or pain during surgery	1	
	Implicit memory/awareness: Not able to be consciously recalled but may affect behaviour or performance at a later time	1	
b	• Anaesthetic with NMB – 1:8000 • Anaesthetic without NMB – 1:136000 • All GA – 1:19000	1 1 1	These values are taken directly from NAP5 (within 1000).
c	• Tachycardia • Hypertension • Sweating • Tear production • Grimacing/movement • Tachypnoea • Coughing • Pupil dilation	3	These signs would indicate that a patient may be under a light plane of anaesthesia or may be aware. Anaesthetists should be aware if the patient is on medication (e.g. beta blockers/NMBs) that may mask these signs. No half marks, so 1 per correct pair.
d	• Isolated forearm technique • Processed EEG (e.g. BIS/entropy) • Raw EEG • MAC concentration • Auditory evoked potentials • Sensory evoked potentials • Lower oesophageal motility	4	Although lower oesophageal motility and the isolated forearm are of academic/historical use, they can still be considered clinically. 1 mark per correct answer.
e	• Drug factors: TIVA • Patient factors: female gender, age (young adults, but not children), obesity, previous awareness under anaesthesia, difficult airway • Speciality: obstetrics, cardiac, thoracic, neurosurgical • Organisational: out of hours, emergencies, junior members of staff	5	1 mark per correct answer. This is a list from NAP5. Be aware: ASA and physical status were not found to be a causative factor.
f	1. A face-to-face meeting with all patients who experience awareness (meeting) 2. Early consultation with a psychologist/psychiatrist to assess flashbacks, nightmares, anxiety and mood (analysis) 3. Active follow-up at 2 weeks to assess impact, and plan for ongoing follow-up and referral (support)	1 1 1	These are part of the NAP5 awareness support pathway, where they are all emphasised heavily.

Awareness is a big topic within the FRCA curriculum and it is important that all anaesthetists have read the outcomes of NAP5 (the national audit project surrounding accidental awareness under anaesthesia). There are a number of risk factors and a good way of splitting these up would be patient vs. surgical vs. organisational. Knowledge of some of the incidence of awareness is also important and is commonly asked.

Hardman, J. and Aitkenhead, A. (2005) Awareness under anaesthesia. *CEACCP*, **5(6):** 183–186.

Kim, M., Fricchione, G. and Akeju, O. (2021) Accidental awareness under general anaesthesia: incidence, risk factors and psychological management. *BJA Education*, **21(4):** 154–161.

Pandit, J., Cook, T., Jonker, W. and O'Sullivan, E. (2013) A national survey of anaesthetists (NAP5 baseline) to estimate an annual incidence of accidental awareness during general anaesthesia in the UK. *British Journal of Anaesthesia*, **110(4):** 501–9.

CRQ 11: answer guidance

Syllabus	EN_IK_10
Question type	Medium: pass mark 12
Topic	**Anaesthesia for children with learning disorders**
Aim	To be able to recall the issues in pre-assessment and pre-operative care for patients with learning disabilities, and how these are overcome.
Pass requirements	List the options for pre-medication of the learning disability patient.

Q	Answer	Marks	Guidance
a	• Difficulty with communication • Difficulty with social interaction • Difficulty with imagination	1 1 1	These are the so-called 'triad of impairments'. Variations in the language can be accepted as a correct answer.
b	• There may be issues surrounding consent for the procedure Patients may: • be unable to describe symptoms • be unable to recall medical history • not tolerate any physical contact during examination • not be able to understand instructions for investigations (e.g. taking a deep breath for a chest X-ray) • have difficulty cooperating with invasive investigations	4	1 mark per correct answer. Parents or guardians will be heavily relied upon for history and investigations; however, there may be gaps in their knowledge, especially if the patient lives in a residential home.

Q	Answer	Marks	Guidance
c	• Pre-assessment can be achieved over the phone • Information gathering prior to admission (e.g. height, weight) • Providing a quiet area for the patient to wait prior to admission • First on the list to prevent prolonged starvation • Patients are encouraged to bring familiar toys and games to calm them • Familiar parent or carer can stay with the patient as long as possible	4	1 mark per correct answer. Each of these will facilitate smooth transition to anaesthetic room. Restraint should be avoided unless undertaken by a trained professional.
d	**To facilitate cannulation:** • Ametop (4%): 1.5g per dose • EMLA (5%): 5g per pack **For sedation:** • Midazolam (PO): 0.25–1.0mg/kg • Ketamine (PO): 3–5mg/kg • Ketamine (IM): 1–2mg/kg • Clonidine (PO): 4mcg/kg • Lorazepam (PO): 50–100mcg/kg **For PONV prophylaxis:** • Ondansetron: 0.1mg/kg • Cyclizine: 0.5–1mg/kg (50mg if >12years)	4	1 mark per correct answer. Candidates should not forget that pre-medications in paediatrics or patients with learning difficulties are not limited to sedatives.
e	• IV cannula or NG tubes may become dislodged quickly post-operatively so will need to be secured • Patients may not be able to verbalise pain • Patients may not be able to operate a PCA if needed • Normal routine will be disrupted, which may exacerbate distress • Areas with wounds or local anaesthetic infiltration may be scratched, bitten or pulled, as it is an abnormal sensation	3	1 mark per correct answer. Can accept anything else reasonable, but these are the main post-operative problems. Distress is usually caused by pain and confusion.
f	• Use of visual aids such as 'symbol selection' • Visual pain scales • Basic sign language/Makaton • Facilitate early return of carer/guardian	2	1 mark per correct answer. There are various tools for communication. The easiest will be to facilitate the early return of a carer who will be able to communicate more easily than staff.

Some degree of learning disability is thought to be present in 2% of the population. In the context of autism spectrum disorder, no two patients are the same. They can have differences in levels of knowledge, understanding, and their ability to change routine. Because of its prevalence, anaesthetists should expect to come into contact with these patients on a regular basis. Most units will have a specified pathway to facilitate surgery in the least distressing manner. They are also likely to have a learning disability specialist nurse, or in some cases a psychologist, who may help. Older patients with severe disease may also benefit from a play specialist or run-throughs prior to the day. Pre-medication in these patients may be important, but so called 'car park' sedation should be avoided unless very experienced or in a specialist unit.

Short, J. and Calder, A. (2013) Anaesthesia for children with special needs including autism spectrum disorder. *CEACCP*, **13(4):** 107–112.

CRQ 12: answer guidance

Syllabus	PR_IK_02
Question type	Moderate: pass mark 12
Topic	**Serotonin syndrome**
Aim	To understand the serotonin metabolism pathway and how drugs can interact with it.
Pass requirements	Know the triad of features that are in keeping with serotonin syndrome.

Q	Answer	Marks	Guidance
a	• Changes in mental status • Neuromuscular abnormalities • Autonomic hyperactivity	1 1 1	These are the typical triad of features. Listing more than one autonomic feature will not gain more than one mark.
b	The patient must have current or previous use of a medication with serotonergic activity	1	This is essential to be able to make a diagnosis.
c	• VBG (as a marker of metabolic acidosis) • LFTs (raised liver enzymes) • U&Es (raised serum creatinine) • FBC (leucocytosis) • Serum creatinine phosphokinase	3	1 mark per correct answer. Other reasonable laboratory tests could be accepted, but these would be the most common.
d	• Malignant hyperthermia • Anticholinergic syndrome • Opiate toxicity • Neuroleptic malignant syndrome • Peri-operative delirium • Sedative-hypnotic withdrawal • Sepsis/infection	4	1 mark per correct answer. Other differentials can be accepted within reason, but at least 3 should be from the list in this table.

Q	Answer	Marks	Guidance
e	**Synthesised:** brainstem raphe nuclei	1	1 mark per correct answer.
	Found in: hypothalamus, thalamus, limbic system, cerebellum, spinal cord, retina, enterochromaffin cells (of the enteric nervous system), platelets, mast cells	3	Must include where it is synthesised to gain maximum marks.
f	7	1	There are 7 classes of receptor.
g	**Enhanced serotonin release:** MDMA, cocaine, fenfluramine, phenylpiperidine opioids (fentanyl and meperidine), oxycodone, tramadol	1	All of these drugs have some activity on the serotonin metabolism pathway. The primary driver of serotonin syndrome is an overload of the amount of serotonin, and therefore any drugs with an effect on the pathway have potential to cause it.
	Serotonin reuptake inhibition: SSRIs (paroxetine, sertraline, citalopram, fluoxetine), SNRIs (venlafaxine and duloxetine), tricyclic antidepressants (amitriptyline, imipramine, clomipramine, desipramine), phenylpiperidine opioids (fentanyl and meperidine), tramadol, ondansetron, granisetron	1	
	Serotonin metabolism: MAOIs (phenelzine, moclobemide, selegiline), methylene blue, hydralazine, linezolid	1	
	Direct agonist: triptans (sumatriptan, rizatriptan, zolmitriptan), ergot alkaloids	1	

As more people are started on antidepressants in the community, it is likely that presentations with serotonin syndrome could increase. It is important for anaesthetists to be aware of the many manifestations, as multiple anaesthetic drugs can have an effect on the serotonin metabolism pathway. Often, these patients need only routine supportive care but could require ICU admission for the initial 24–48 hours. There are no definitive treatments.

Bartakke, J., Corredor, C. and van Rensburg, A. (2020) Serotonin syndrome in the perioperative period. *BJA Education*, **20(1):** 10–17.

SBA 1: answer = D – CT venogram of head

This patient has the symptoms of venous sinus thrombosis, a rare but possible post-partum complication. Risk factors for this condition include being dehydrated, anaemic and having a caesarean section. Tension headache or PDPH are the most common headaches post delivery, but this patient having some blurred vision and the course of the headache, as well as the aforementioned risk factors, point towards venous sinus thrombosis. The most appropriate investigation for this would be a CT venogram.

Kearsley, R. and Stocks, G. (2020) Venous thromboembolism in pregnancy – diagnosis, management and treatment. *BJA Education*, **21(3):** 117–123.

Liang, Z., Gao, W. and Feng, L. (2017) Clinical characteristics and prognosis of cerebral venous thrombosis in Chinese women during pregnancy and puerperium. *Nature Scientific Reports*, **7:** 43866.

SBA 2: answer = D – Central core myopathy

The only two neuromuscular conditions thought to be linked to MH are central core myopathy and familial periodic paralysis. Duchenne muscular dystrophy and to a lesser extent Becker muscular dystrophy are thought to be a risk of anaesthetic-induced rhabdomyolysis (AIR). This is a condition with a similar constellation of signs and symptoms.

Marsh, S., Ross, N. and Pittard, A. (2011) Neuromuscular disorders and anaesthesia. Part 1: generic anaesthetic management. *CEACCP*, **11(4):** 115–118.

Marsh, S. and Pittard, A. (2011) Neuromuscular disorders and anaesthesia. Part 2: specific neuromuscular disorders. *CEACCP*, **11(4):** 119–123.

SBA 3: answer = E – Single lung lavage in cystic fibrosis

There are three broad absolute indications for one-lung ventilation:
- to prevent damage or contamination to healthy lung (such as lung abscess and pulmonary haemorrhage)
- to control distribution of ventilation (such as bronchopleural fistula and traumatic bronchial disruption)
- to facilitate single lung lavage (such as in cystic fibrosis or pulmonary alveolar proteinosis).

All others are relative indications, but one-lung ventilation is frequently used.

Ashok, V. and Francis, J. (2018) A practical approach to adult one-lung ventilation. *BJA Education*, **18(3):** 69–74.

SBA 4: answer = C – Infraclavicular block

Surgery of the upper limb is a common indication for the use of regional anaesthesia. Direct block of the ulnar nerve is the most inappropriate block to use, as there is likely to be some anatomical areas missed and a higher likelihood the block will fail. For this type of surgery it is likely the surgeons will use a tourniquet and therefore it is prudent to pick a block that will cover this. The interscalene block often has inconsistent blockade of the lower trunk and higher risk of phrenic nerve palsy, which may affect discharge. The supraclavicular block has a higher risk of pneumothorax than the infraclavicular block and so the latter would be used preferentially. The axillary block, whilst similarly efficacious, would potentially require more punctures and so may confer increased risk of nerve damage or bleeding.

Mirza, F. and Brown, A. (2011) Ultrasound-guided regional anaesthesia for procedures of the upper extremity. *Anaesthesiology Research and Practice*, **579824:** 1–6.

SBA 5: answer = C – The thoracic paravertebral sympathetic chain consists of ganglia from T1–T7

The autonomic nervous system is divided into the sympathetic and parasympathetic nervous system. The sympathetic nervous system originates from the grey matter of the lateral horn of the spinal cord from T1 to L2/3. The paravertebral sympathetic chain is divided into 4 parts (cervical, thoracic, lumbar and pelvic plexuses). The thoracic portion consists of a series of ganglia from T1–T5. The parasympathetic system originates from cranial nerves 3, 7, 9 and 10, as well as fibres from the ventral rami of S2–S4. Preganglionic fibres are myelinated and postganglionic fibres are unmyelinated but whether they are part of the parasympathetic or sympathetic nervous system depends on the length of those fibres, with few exceptions.

Bankenahally, R. and Krovvidi, H. (2016) Autonomic nervous system: anatomy, physiology and relevance in anaesthesia and critical care medicine. *BJA Education*, **16(11):** 381–387.

SBA 6: answer = E – Commence CPR

The patient is in anaphylaxis and their blood pressure has dropped to below 50mmHg. This fulfils the criteria of starting CPR immediately and declaring a cardiac arrest as per AAGBI guidelines. Whilst adrenaline is a key part of the management of anaphylaxis, at this point the blood pressure alone would mean CPR rather than drug management. Hydrocortisone has no role in the immediate management in this case and although the patient should receive fluids, CPR is the most important treatment strategy.

Association of Anaesthetists of Great Britain and Ireland (2021) *Anaphylaxis Quick Reference Guide: version 4.*

SBA 7: answer = B – Aspirate with 16–18G cannula

This is a secondary pneumothorax due to the patient's heavy smoking history and thus warrants treatment rather than observation or repeat chest X-ray. Following the British Thoracic Society guidelines, this pneumothorax should be aspirated with a 16–18G cannula. A chest drain of either Seldinger or surgical type is not required immediately; however, if there is no resolution of the pneumothorax with aspiration, a chest drain will be necessary.

Macduff, A. (2010) Management of spontaneous pneumothorax: British Thoracic Society pleural disease guideline 2010. *Thorax*, **supp2(ii):** 18–31.

SBA 8: answer = B – White ethnicity

Many risk factors have been identified for pyloric stenosis; however, of the options presented, only white ethnicity increases risk. It is more prevalent in male infants (4:1 ratio), those born at term, first-born infants, bottle-fed infants, those born by caesarean section and those born in autumn or spring, but the causation of some of these associations cannot be established. There is a probable genetic component as it is more common in those with affected parents, and it has a high concordance in monozygotic twins. While *Helicobacter pylori* infection has been proposed as a potential causative agent, there is no evidence that maternal infection with *H. pylori* increases risk.

Fell, D. and Chelliah, S. (2001) Infantile pyloric stenosis. *British Journal of Anaesthesia CEPD Reviews*, **1(3):** 85–88.

Zhu, J., Zhu, T., Lin, Z., Qu, Y. and Mu, D. (2017) Perinatal risk factors for infantile hypertrophic pyloric stenosis: a meta-analysis. *Journal of Pediatric Surgery*, **52(9):** 1389–1397.

SBA 9: answer = A – Femoral and popliteal block with perineural catheters inserted and post-operative infusion of local anaesthetic

Phantom limb pain and stump pain are particularly troublesome following an amputation and can lead to increased morbidity. In the initial post-operative phase stump pain predominates, with phantom limb pain taking over after this. If presented with a patient in acute stump pain post-operatively it would be reasonable to prescribe opiates or commence an opiate PCA, but ideally the management of these patients would be to prevent this from occurring. The ideal way to facilitate this would be through good perineural blockade, which can attenuate peripheral and central sensitisation. Siting an epidural would be associated with more complications and a spinal anaesthetic will only really be useful up to 24 hours post-operatively. Lidocaine may have some use but as yet this is an unestablished treatment strategy.

Neil, M. (2016) Pain after amputation. *BJA Education*, **16(3):** 107–112.

SBA 10: answer = E – Polycythaemia rubra vera

Advanced age is not a contraindication to free-flap microsurgery. While smoking and obesity do indeed affect the success of the surgery in question, they are relative contraindications. Patients are recommended to stop smoking for 4 weeks, and if obese, to commence a weight management programme. Sickle cell trait has reduced features compared to sickle cell disease, and is therefore not an absolute contraindication. Polycythaemia and other hypercoagulable states result in failure due to anastomotic thrombosis.

Nimalan, N., Alexandre Branford, O. and Stocks, G. (2016) Anaesthesia for free flap breast reconstruction. *BJA Education*, **16(5):** 162–166.

SBA 11: answer = E – Gastro-oesophageal reflux

Gastro-oesophageal reflux is the most common post-operative complication and can affect 35–58% of patients undergoing a corrective procedure. This is likely due to intrinsic oesophageal dysfunction. All the other options are possible but are less common than GORD. Most patients will remain on prophylactic antibiotics to reduce the risk of post-operative chest infection. Anastomotic leak occurs in 11–21% of patients and of these, 50% develop a stricture. Tracheomalacia occurs due to the trachea retaining a wide membranous section rather than its normal C shape.

Al-Rawi, O. and Booker, P. (2017) Oeosophageal atresia and tracheo-oesophageal fistula. *CEACCP*, **7(1):** 15–19.

SBA 12: answer = D – Ropivacaine – 8.1

The dissociation of local anaesthetic is determined by the pH of the local tissue and the pKa of the drug. The pKa is the pH at which 50% of the local anaesthetic is ionised and 50% is unionised. Local anaesthetics with a lower pKa have a faster onset of action: this is due to the fact that a larger proportion of the drug is in its unionised form. The correct pKa values are as follows: lidocaine (7.8), bupivacaine (8.1), prilocaine (7.7), ropivacaine (8.1) and cocaine (8.6). All of these local anaesthetics are in common use for clinical practice so it is important to be able to compare their physical characteristics to clinical action.

Taylor, A. and McLeod, G. (2014) Basic pharmacology of local anaesthetics. *BJA Education*, **20(2):** 34–41.

SBA 13: answer = B – Immediate intubation and ventilation and monitor patient in the operating theatre

This patient has a total spinal due to an intrathecal dose of the anaesthetic low dose mix. The fact that the patient has difficulty in breathing would suggest that she is now compromised and so would require intubation and ventilation. If the CTG remains normal, then a possible option would be to wait rather than rush for a caesarean section (putting mother and baby at further risk). However, this would need discussion with both a senior anaesthetist and obstetrician. Removing the catheter at this point would not be useful. Although further resuscitation may be required, control of ventilation and oxygenation takes priority. The patient has not shown signs of local anaesthetic toxicity so intralipid is not indicated.

Desai, N. and Carvalho, B. (2021) Conversion of labour epidural analgesia to surgical anaesthesia for emergency intrapartum Caesarean section. *BJA Education*, **20(1):** 213–219.

SBA 14: answer = E – Neck irradiation

Difficult face mask ventilation is noted in approximately 5% of all patients. The key causes for it are identified as obesity, bearded, elderly, snorer, edentulous, males, limited jaw protrusion, Mallampati 3 or 4, and neck irradiation. Of those, neck irradiation is the most significant.

Crawley, S. and Dalton, A. (2015) Predicting the difficult airway. *BJA Education*, **15(5):** 253–257.

SBA 15: answer = B – CHADS$_2$ score >3

The following have been identified as having a higher risk of peri-procedural stroke: recent TIA/stroke, CHADS$_2$ score >3, mechanical heart valves and rheumatic heart disease.

Lindberg, A. and Flexman, A. (2021) Perioperative stroke after non-cardiac, non-neurological surgery. *BJA Education*, **21(2):** 59–65.

SBA 16: answer = E – Carbamazepine

All treatments other than carbamazepine are first-line for neuropathic limb pain; second-line being any other of the 4 agents. Carbamazepine is first-line treatment for trigeminal neuralgia.

NICE (2013, updated 2020) *Neuropathic pain in adults* [CG173]. Available at: www.nice.org.uk/guidance/cg173 (accessed 24 January 2022)

SBA 17: answer = A – Further fluid bolus 20ml/kg

This patient has presented with signs of shock, most likely as a result of bacterial meningitis. Initial therapy should include fluid resuscitation: 3 boluses of 20ml/kg is recommended, followed by early instigation of vasopressor therapy. In this case, the patient has had 2 boluses of fluid as per APLS guidance (the patient's weight is approximately 18kg) and so they should have a further bolus of 360ml balanced crystalloid. Following this IV dopamine would be the vasopressor of choice. These patients can decompensate rapidly so intubation and ventilation could be indicated, but it would not be advisable to do this until the patient has been adequately resuscitated. IV phenylephrine has no role in management here, nor do central access and noradrenaline infusion in the acute phase.

O'Reilly, H. and Menon, K. (2021) Sepsis in paediatrics. *BJA Education*, **21(2):** 51–58.

SBA 18: answer = B – IV rasburicase

Tumour lysis syndrome (combined with the features described) may also include hyperphosphataemia and hypocalcaemia, as well as increased serum and urine uric acid. The first line of management is aggressive fluid resuscitation, treatment of hyperkalaemia and administration of rasburicase. If the patient does not improve then they may require CVVHF. Allopurinol or rasburicase can be given prophylactically in those who are at increased risk due to higher grade lymphomas. Forced alkaline diuresis has variable efficacy. Bicarbonate will only give temporary improvement to the patient's pH but does not address the underlying issue.

Beed, M., Levitt, M. and Bokari, S. (2010) Intensive care management of patients with haematological malignancy. *CEACCP*, **10(6):** 167–171.

SBA 19: answer = D – Open surgery (vs. laparoscopic surgery)

Phaeochromocytoma, although rare, requires specific anaesthetic management. The anaesthetic approach should favour techniques that will avoid large changes in blood pressure intra-operatively. There are a number of risk factors for intra-operative haemodynamic instability, including size of the tumour, pre-induction MAP >100mmHg, high pre-operative plasma noradrenaline levels and postural drop following alpha blockade. There is no evidence to favour one surgical approach over another in terms of instability, but laparoscopic surgery does favour reduced recovery times.

Connor, D. and Boumphrey, S. (2016) Perioperative care of phaeochromocytoma. *BJA Education*, **16(5):** 153–158.

SBA 20: answer = B – Intrathoracic pressure is suddenly released and associated pooling of blood in pulmonary vessels causes a drop in BP

The Valsalva manoeuvre can be useful in the treatment of supraventricular tachycardias and in the diagnosis of autonomic dysfunction. It follows 4 main phases: increase in intrathoracic pressure, reduced venous return and baroreceptor reflex, sudden drop in intrathoracic pressure then overshoot.

Kumar, C. and Van Zundert, A. (2018) Intraoperative Valsalva maneuver: a narrative review. *Canadian Journal of Anesthesia*, **65(5):** 578–585.

SBA 21: answer = D – Phrenic nerve palsy

Phrenic nerve palsy is a known complication of an interscalene block, which would have been the block of choice for shoulder replacement surgery. This can make the patient short of breath but is usually self-limiting, and respiratory function will recover when the block wears off. If the patient decompensates, they may need high flow nasal oxygen or CPAP until full recovery. Inadequate reversal and opiate toxicity are possibilities, but are less likely than phrenic nerve palsy, which has an incidence of >80% when using moderate volumes of LA. Post-operative anxiety and MI are less likely.

Hewson, D., Oldman, M. and Bedforth, N. (2019) Regional anaesthesia for shoulder surgery. *BJA Education*, **19(4):** 98–104.

SBA 22: answer = B – In the anaesthetic room prior to induction

The ICD should be turned off in the anaesthetic room where there is a high level of monitoring and before any intervention has taken place. Deactivating too early (pre-operatively in day surgery ward) opens the patient to possible arrhythmia and arrest pre-surgery. Post-induction may be too late; some anaesthetic drugs can be pro-arrhythmogenic. The use of surgical diathermy increases risk of damage to the ICD and triggering arrhythmia intra-operatively. The ICD should be turned on as soon as possible following surgery; and while the ICD is not active, the patient should have defibrillator pads on their chest wall ready to treat any arrhythmia.

Bryant, H., Roberts, P. and Diprose, P. (2016) Perioperative management of patients with cardiac implantable electronic devices. *BJA Education*, **16(11):** 388–396.

SBA 23: answer = E – No anaesthesia required

This patient has a history of complete cord transection with associated loss of sensation. Considering the patient has had previous anaesthesia without any issue, the risk of autonomic dysreflexia is low. Therefore it may be appropriate to have an anaesthetist on standby but without the need for the anaesthetic itself. Neuraxial block may be challenging in these patients due to difficulties with positioning and the presence of contractures. General anaesthesia may not be required unless there are significant risk factors.

Petsas, A. and Drake, J. (2015) Perioperative management for patients with a chronic spinal cord injury. *BJA Education*, **15(3):** 123–130.

SBA 24: answer = D – Chi-squared test

The data presented is an example of discrete categorical data and therefore the only appropriate statistical test would be the chi-squared test. All the other tests listed are for continuous data and would therefore be inappropriate in this case.

McCluskey, A. and Lalkhen, A. (2008) Statistics III: probability and statistical tests. *CEACCP*, **7(5):** 167–170.

SBA 25: answer = C – Tension headache

The most common form of headache in new mothers is a simple tension headache, which usually resolves with simple analgesia and rest. The typical symptom is a band-like headache with no focal neurology. Migraine is also a possibility, especially if the woman is known to have migraines, but this would be associated with auras. Cluster headaches are a rarer type of headache and less likely. The risk of a PDPH from an uncomplicated spinal anaesthetic is low, and it is therefore less likely to be the cause of a headache compared to a simple tension headache. If the patient has a history of pre-eclampsia or eclampsia, this would prompt investigation for subarachnoid haemorrhage, but this patient lacks those risk factors.

Sabharwal, A. and Stocks, G. (2011) Post-partum headache: diagnosis and management. *CEACCP*, **11(5):** 181–185.

SBA 26: answer = A – Central cord syndrome

These findings are typical of central cord syndrome, which can be caused by severe hyperextension of the neck. Patients with arthritis are more likely to develop central cord syndrome due to exacerbation of long-standing cervical spondylosis when the neck is hyperextended. It is a partial lesion of the spinal cord and is associated with a more favourable prognosis than other spinal cord injuries. Patients may also develop urinary retention. The sensory loss in central cord syndrome is variable. These symptoms could be present in electrolyte imbalance or infarction, but the bilateral upper limb deficit makes it more likely to be central cord syndrome. Peripheral nerve injury would be more likely to affect a single nerve rather than causing bilateral symptoms.

Bonner, S. and Smith, C. (2013) Initial management of acute spinal cord injury. *CEACCP*, **13(6):** 224–231.

SBA 27: answer = E – Maintain forward flow of blood through the heart

For regurgitant lesions, the haemodynamic goal should be to maintain forward flow. Anything that increases afterload – especially on the left side of the heart – will result in an increase of the regurgitant fraction. Use of high doses of vasopressors should be avoided because of this.

Chacko, M. and Weinberg, J. (2012) Aortic valve stenosis: perioperative anaesthetic implications of surgical replacement and minimally invasive interventions. *CEACCP*, **(12)6:** 295–301.

SBA 28: answer = B – Inadvertent femoral nerve block

Inadvertent femoral nerve block is a known complication of ilioinguinal nerve block, especially if it has not been performed using ultrasound guidance. This is usually self-limiting and does not preclude the patient from being discharged home. The second most likely scenario would be poor positioning causing nerve damage. Damage to the ilioinguinal nerve is unlikely to cause any motor weakness; the same can be said for the sciatic nerve.

Lipp, A., Woodcock, J., Hensman, B. and Wilkinson, K. (2004) Leg weakness is a complication of ilioinguinal nerve block in children. *British Journal of Anaesthesia*, **92(2):** 273–274.

SBA 29: answer = A – Venous drainage is via 1 anterior and 2 posterior spinal veins

The venous drainage of the spinal cord is from 3 anterior and 3 posterior veins which form a valveless anastomotic network on the surface of the spinal cord. This drains into internal and external plexuses. The other options are all correct. It is important to understand the arterial supply of the vertebral system, as this can lead to different clinical pictures if disrupted.

Bonner, S. and Smith, C. (2013) Initial management of acute spinal cord injury. *CEACCP*, **13(6):** 224–231.

SBA 30: answer = C – 7 size E cylinders

The total volume of oxygen which will be consumed by the patient on the journey will be 2100L. This is calculated by [(rr × tv × 0.5) + 500] × 10. It is recommended to take twice the total volume needed to complete the journey. The sizes of cylinders are as follows:
- Size D: 340L
- Size E: 680L
- Size F: 1360L.

Therefore the ideal number and size of cylinder to take would be 7 size E cylinders.

Bourn, S., Wijesingha, S. and Nordmann, G. (2017) Transfer of the critically ill adult patient. *BJA Education*, **18(3):** 63–68.

SBA 31: answer = C – Driving pressure

The driving pressure is the most influential changeable variable for CO_2 elimination in jet ventilation. This changes tidal volume and therefore inspired and expired CO_2. Increasing frequency may in fact reduce CO_2 elimination by reducing the tidal volume. Inspiratory time and expiratory time have no influence independently on CO_2 elimination. Peak airway pressure is not a variable that can be directly measured in this mode.

Evans, E., Biro, P. and Bedforth, N. (2007) Jet ventilation. *CEACCP*, **7(1):** 2–5.

SBA 32: answer = B – Type II endoleak

The radiologist is describing a type II endoleak, where the patient's aneurysm sac is being filled by a branch vessel. Type II endoleaks are common after surgery (10–25%); the significance remains debatable. The management of these would be by routine surveillance. Type I (graft seal failure) and type III (leak through graft fabric) endoleaks are less common. In these cases it is reasonable to complete the EVAR procedure and consider open surgery at a later date. Type IV endoleaks are due to porosity in the graft itself and usually intentional. There are no type V endoleaks.

Kasipandian, V. and Pichel, A. (2012) Complex endovascular aortic aneurysm repair. *CEACCP*, **(12)6:** 312–316.

SBA 33: answer = D – Opioid-induced hyperalgesia

OIH is the decrease in nociceptive threshold caused by exposure to opioids. If mistaken for tolerance, and an opioid dose is increased, the pain induced is typically worsened. The exact mechanism for this phenomenon has yet to be fully elucidated, but some central pathways have been implicated.

Gallagher, H. and Galvin, D. (2018) Opioids for chronic non-cancer use. *BJA Education*, **18(11):** 337–341.

SBA 34: answer = D – Ask for a child safeguarding lead to attend theatre

This is a difficult situation as there could be a serious safeguarding issue. There may also be other vulnerable children or adults in the same household that may be in immediate danger. As the child is already under anaesthesia, it is more prudent to continue with the surgery. However, the Trust safeguarding lead for children should attend as soon as possible to carry out a full investigation and examination before proceeding. Interviewing the parent alone could lead to personal danger, but also more danger to any possible vulnerable adults or children, as well as legal issues. Taking photographs may be useful, but should only be done in combination with the safeguarding lead.

Melarkode, K. and Wilkinson, K. (2012) Child protection and the anaesthetist. *CEACCP*, **12(3):** 123–127.

SBA 35: answer = C – Ethambutol

Ethambutol is the most commonly implicated drug for visual disturbance in TB treatment. It is generally well tolerated; however, it can cause visual disturbance and loss of colour vision. If this occurs it should be stopped and triple therapy continued on the advice of the local TB specialist.

Bashford, T. and Howell, V. (2018) Tropical medicine and anaesthesia 1. *BJA Education*, **18(2):** 35–40.

SBA 36: answer = D – Use of mild sedation

The national consensus, supported by *WHO surgical safety checklist supporting information* (2009) is that the only mark on the patient should be placed by the surgical team. Any additional mark placed in relation to the block risks introducing error. Although the debate continues surrounding use of sedation for blocks, mild sedation, which maintains verbal contact with the patient, is less likely to introduce error in this situation.

Topor, B., Oldman, M. and Nicholls, B. (2020) Best practices for safety and quality in peripheral regional anaesthesia. *BJA Education*, **20(10):** 341–347.

SBA 37: answer = A – Chromosome 19

Chromosome 19 contains the susceptibility locus for the defective type-1 ryanodine receptor calcium-release channel. This causes unregulated release of calcium when uncoupling is triggered by volatile anaesthetic agents and depolarising neuromuscular blockade. Early recognition of these patients is of critical importance, and management will include rapid treatment with dantrolene, removal of the causative agent and active cooling.

Rosenberg, H., Pollock, N., Schiemann, A., Bulger, T. and Stowell, K. (2015) Malignant hyperthermia: a review. *Orphanet Journal of Rare Diseases*, **10(1):** 93.

SBA 38: answer = C – IV MgSO$_4$ 4g

This patient is having an eclamptic seizure and so the immediate management would be a bolus of magnesium sulfate followed by an infusion. If this doesn't terminate the seizure, a further bolus of magnesium sulfate can be given. Intravenous benzodiazepines can be given to terminate seizures but these are not first-line. The same applies for intravenous phenytoin or levetiracetam.

Leslie, D. and Collis, R. (2016) Hypertension in pregnancy. *BJA Education*, **16(1)**: 33–37.

SBA 39: answer = E – IV dexamethasone 6.6mg

The patient has a large brain tumour and signs of raised intracranial pressure. Treatment should be focused on reducing the ICP and early assessment by a neurosurgeon. Steroids are useful in reducing neurogenic oedema so should be first line; however, this can be combined with hypertonic saline. Mannitol should only be used after discussion with the neurosurgical team or second line. Furthermore the doses for both are incorrect. Lorazepam is not likely to be of benefit if the patient is already adequately sedated. IV acetazolamide is not in the treatment algorithm for raised ICP and will be too slow to work effectively. The patient should be kept sedated and ventilation parameters as per head trauma.

Young, A. and Marsh, S. (2018) Steroid use in critical care. *BJA Education*, **18(5)**: 129–134.

SBA 40: answer = B – Milrinone

This patient needs to receive an inotrope to improve contractility of the heart and facilitate coming off cardiopulmonary bypass. This can be achieved with drugs like dobutamine and milrinone as first-line agents. Milrinone is also a potent pulmonary vasodilator and is indicated if there are signs of pulmonary hypertension.

St André, A. and DelRossi, A. (2005) Hemodynamic management of patients in the first 24 hours after cardiac surgery. *Critical Care Medicine*, **(33)9**: 2082–2093.

SBA 41: answer = A – Posterior tibial nerve

The deep ventral structures, muscles and the sole of the foot are innervated by the posterior tibial nerve, which is a branch of the tibial nerve. The sural nerve innervates the lateral aspect of the foot. The calcaneal nerve supplies the posterior aspect of the foot. The deep peroneal nerve supplies the webspace between the first and second toes and the superficial peroneal nerve supplies the dorsum of the foot.

Purushothaman, L., Allan, A. and Bedforth, N. (2013) Ultrasound-guided ankle block. *BJA Education*, **13(5)**: 174–178.

SBA 42: answer = B – 30ml/min/100g of tissue

The resting splanchnic blood flow is 30ml/min/100g of tissue, which equates to 25–30% of the cardiac output. It can decrease to <10ml/min/100g in low cardiac output states, but can also increase to 250ml/min/100g after a large meal. The blood flow is maintained via auto-regulation intrinsically, extrinsically and via the humeral system.

Harper, D. and Chandler, B. (2016) Splanchnic circulation. *BJA Education*, **16(2)**: 66–71.

SBA 43: answer = E – Open strap muscles with surgical scissors

This is both an anaesthetic and surgical emergency. Management of this patient is with the 'SCOOP' approach (skin exposure, cut sutures, open skin, open strap muscles and pack wound) followed by immediate transfer to theatre. A scalpel thyroidotomy is likely to be complex and unsuccessful on the ward and should only be attempted as a last resort. Intubation on the ward may be challenging, as anatomy may be significantly distorted. There may not be time to transfer the patient to theatre at this point without an attempt to relieve some airway obstruction. High flow nasal oxygen will be of little benefit here due to an obstructing trachea.

El-Boghdadly, K. (2021) Management of haematoma after thyroid surgery: systematic review and multidisciplinary consensus guidelines from the Difficult Airway Society, the British Association of Endocrine and Thyroid Surgeons and the British Association of Otorhinolaryngology, Head and Neck Surgery. *Anaesthesia Guidelines*, 15585.

SBA 44: answer = C – Aim to keep haemoglobin >70g/L

Fluid and blood product management is crucial during vascular surgery. For AAA repair, most patients have concurrent ischaemic heart disease, thus requiring a higher transfusion threshold of 90g/L. Fluids are crucial to prevent hypotension after aortic unclamping, with both colloids and crystalloids suitable to keep CVP >12–15mmHg.

Al-Hashimi, M. and Thompson, J. (2013) Anaesthesia for elective open abdominal aortic aneurysm repair. *CEACCP*, **13(6):** 208–212.

SBA 45: answer = C – Peripheral venepuncture

The *Europain study 2014* focused on pain scores for procedures on the ICU. Peripheral venepuncture was found to be the least painful procedure of all those experienced by patients in the ICU, with removal of chest tubes and surgical drains being the most painful.

Puntillo, K., Max, A., Timsit, J.-F. *et al.* (2014) Determinants of procedural pain intensity in the intensive care unit. The Europain® study. *American Journal of Respiratory Critical Care Medicine*, **189(1):** 39–47.

SBA 46: answer = C – 12.5mg

The correct dose of oral midazolam for conscious sedation is 0.5mg/kg. This can be added to some strong-tasting fruit squash or sugary drink to facilitate the taking of the medication, as it can taste very bitter. Other options for conscious sedation could be ketamine 5–10mg/kg IM. Nitrous oxide can also be used but is likely to be less reliable.

Sury, M. (2012) Conscious sedation in children. *CEACCP*, **12(3):** 152–156.

SBA 47: answer = E – Commence infusion of vasopressin and titrate as required

The patient is unresponsive to IV fluid therapy and has now gone into vasodilatory shock. The first-line treatment for brainstem-dead patients awaiting donation is vasopressin. Whilst other vasopressors may be used, vasopressin may also have some benefit in the treatment of central diabetes insipidus. Continued fluid therapy in refractory vasodilation may cause pulmonary oedema and hypoxia.

Corbett, S., Trainor, D. and Gaffney, A. (2021) Perioperative management of the organ donor after diagnosis of death using neurological criteria. *BJA Education*, **21(5):** 194–200.

SBA 48: answer = E – Age >50

According to NICE guidance, patients aged over 60 years are associated with an increased risk of VTE, which would therefore require prophylactic treatment. All other options are risk factors and would require prophylaxis. This information is normally listed on any inpatient drug chart. There are also important exclusion criteria for the use of VTE prophylaxis that one should be familiar with in the pre-operative phase.

NICE (2010) *Venous thromboembolism: reducing the risk of venous thromboembolism (deep vein thrombosis and pulmonary embolism) in patients admitted to hospital* [CG92].

SBA 49: answer = D – Predominantly in non-dependent lung (dorsal)

When the patient is proned and ventilated, the predominant area of ventilation is in the dorsal region of the non-dependent lung. If the patient were not mechanically ventilated, then ventilation across the lung would be more uniform in nature. Proning a patient with respiratory disease can be a useful strategy to reduce the V/Q mismatch and may improve oxygenation.

Lumb, A. and White, A. (2021) Breathing in the prone position in health and disease. *BJA Education*, **21(8):** 280–283.

SBA 50: answer = C – Baseline at 160bpm, variability 30bpm, variable decelerations with no concerning characteristics for 90 minutes

The accepted normal range for the CTG baseline is 110–160bpm. Variability of the baseline of <5 or >25 is considered abnormal. Decelerations are judged as being non-concerning or concerning, based on their pattern (early/late). Despite showing no concerning characteristics, variable decelerations for ≥90 minutes indicates an abnormal trace.

Jayasooriya, G. and Djapardy, V. (2017) Intrapartum assessment of fetal well-being. *BJA Education*, **17(12):** 406–411.

SBA 51: answer = B – Chest X-ray

Expiratory stridor is a sign of tracheal obstruction. There could be an extrinsic mass causing compression, such as a retrosternal goitre. Higher obstructions in the oropharynx cause snoring and gurgling. Base of tongue and glottis obstruction cause an inspiratory stridor and dyspnoea, and can cause paroxysmal nocturnal dyspnoea. A chest X-ray can be performed easily and quickly and may show a variety of airway pathologies, including retrosternal goitre. Further airway evaluation is likely to be needed after this.

Lynch, J. and Crawley, S. (2018) Management of airway obstruction. *BJA Education*, **18(2):** 46–51.

SBA 52: answer = A – 0.5% proxymetacaine eye drops

Topicalisation of the eye prior to instrumentation during the sub-Tenon's block is done by blocking trigeminal nerve root terminals in the cornea and conjunctiva. The typical local anaesthetic concentrations used are: 0.5% proxymetacaine, 0.5% tetracaine, 3.5% lidocaine – all used topically as eye drops. Proxymetacaine is preferred as it causes less stinging and is better tolerated.

Anker, R. and Kaur, N. (2017) Regional anaesthesia for ophthalmic surgery. *BJA Education*, **17(7):** 221–227.

SBA 53: answer = C – Pethidine

Pethidine is contraindicated as a first-line choice for management of painful sickle crises, unless specifically detailed in a patient's individual care plan. Painful crises should be treated as a medical emergency. Analgesia must be administered within 30 minutes of presentation to the hospital. Effectiveness of pain relief should be reassessed every 30 minutes as a minimum.

NICE (2012) *Sickle cell disease: managing acute painful episodes in hospital* [CG143]. Available at: www.nice.org.uk/guidance/cg143 (accessed 24 January 2022)

SBA 54: answer = C – Methylene blue

The patient has methaemoglobinaemia, precipitated by prilocaine in the EMLA cream. This gives rise to the classical 'saturation gap', where the patient appears cyanotic despite 100% oxygen and a normal PaO_2. Methaemoglobinaemia may be self-limiting, but the treatment of choice should be methylene blue 1–2mg/kg over 5 minutes. Exchange transfusion, riboflavin and hyperbaric oxygen therapy can be used, but shouldn't be used in the first instance. Prostaglandin infusion is only useful in patients with cyanotic congenital heart disease, which would be corrected before age 5.

Tandale, S., Dave, N. and Garasia, M. (2013) Methemoglobinemia: what the anaesthetist must know. *Indian Journal of Anaesthesia*, **57(4):** 427–428.

SBA 55: answer = A – Further IV fluid bolus of isotonic solution

The patient is clinically hypovolaemic as per the cardiac output studies. The end-diastolic index is low, the extravascular lung water is normal, and the vascular resistance index is within normal range. The first choice of treatment, therefore, is a further bolus of fluid rather than any vasopressors/inotropes. The SVRI being within normal range would suggest limited use for vasopressors at this time.

Drummond, K. and Murphy, E. (2011) Minimally invasive cardiac output monitors. *CEACCP*, **12(1):** 5–10.

SBA 56: answer = D – Smoking causes a rightward shift in the oxygen haemoglobin dissociation curve

Smoking is a modifiable risk factor for many cardiovascular and respiratory diseases, and has a negative effect on other organ systems. It increases the risk of lung cancer, peripheral vascular disease, stroke (including haemorrhagic) and ischaemic heart disease. Cigarettes contain many substances but the addictive component is nicotine, which has a half-life of 30 minutes. It is an inducer of CYP2E1 enzyme activity, which explains smoking's anti-emetic effect. It also results in increased metabolism of volatile anaesthetic agents. Smoking causes a leftward shift in the oxygen–haemoglobin dissociation curve, rather than rightward.

Carrick, M., Robson, J. and Thomas, C. (2019) Smoking and anaesthesia. *BJA Education*, **19(1):** 1–6.

SBA 57: answer = B – 75%

The 'train-of-four' is used to determine receptor occupancy by neuromuscular blockers at the neuromuscular junction. When no twitches are present there is 100% occupation of the receptors. One twitch is equal to 90%, 2 twitches 80%, 3 twitches 75% and 4 twitches <75%. It is important to remember that there needs to be a high degree of occupancy by blocking agents to achieve a clinical effect.

McGrath, C. and Hunter, J. (2006) Monitoring neuromuscular block. *CEACCP*, **6(1):** 7–12.

SBA 58: answer = C – Intercostal

With regard to toxicity, the site of regional anaesthetic block is important. Some sites may carry a higher risk of intravascular injection, such as the stellate ganglion block; others carry an increased risk of rapid absorption due to being in an area of increased vascularity. The highest risk of this is in the intercostal area.

Christie, L., Picard, J. and Weinberg, G. (2015) Local anaesthetic systemic toxicity. *BJA Education*, **15(3):** 136–142.

SBA 59: answer = C – 480s

The administration of heparin prior to vascular catheterisation for cardiopulmonary bypass is essential to prevent fatal thromboembolism. Heparin is usually given at a dose of 300–400IU/kg to achieve an activated clotting time of >480s.

Machin, D. and Allsager, C. (2006) Principles of cardiopulmonary bypass. *CEACCP*, **6(5):** 176–181.

SBA 60: answer = A – Diabetes insipidus

Following pituitary surgery, diabetes insipidus can develop within the first 24 hours and usually spontaneously resolves within 7 days. These patients need supportive management and occasionally require administration of desmopressin. Typically there are no large fluid shifts in neurosurgery, so large volumes of fluid are not given intra-operatively. The stress response to surgery is usually low in pituitary surgery and can be attenuated using intra-operative opiates. An Addisonian crisis would present with a low sodium level and SIADH is unlikely in this clinical scenario.

Menon, R., Murphy, P. and Lindley, A. (2011) Anaesthesia and pituitary disease. *CEACCP*, **11(4):** 133–137.

Practice Paper 2

CRQ 1: Brainstem death and testing

You review a 56-year-old man in the ICU who has had a catastrophic subarachnoid haemorrhage. He is suspected to have brainstem death as a result.

a What are the preconditions that must be fulfilled before brainstem death testing can be undertaken? (4 marks)

i. ....

ii. ....

iii. ....

iv. ....

b Complete the table below regarding brainstem death tests: the cranial nerves involved (3 marks) and the respective methods for testing function (3 marks)

Test	Sensory nerve (S) and Motor nerve (M)	Method for testing function
Pupillary response	S: .... M:	
Ocular-vestibular reflex	S: .... M:	
Response to pain	S: .... M:	

c Which endocrine or hormonal-based treatments may be necessary to correct physiological derangements and support patients for organ donation physiologically, and why? (3 marks)

i. ....

ii. ....

iii. ....

d Describe the cardiovascular response following foramen magnum herniation. (4 marks)

....

....

....

....

e List three contraindications to organ donation. (3 marks)

i. ....

ii. ....

iii. ....

CRQ 2: Spinal cord trauma and autonomic dysreflexia

You are responding to a trauma call in the ED of a district general hospital. A 34-year-old man has been brought in by ambulance after a high-impact road traffic accident. He was reported to be unconscious and immobile at the scene, but was maintaining his airway. He has been transferred with head blocks and his spine has been immobilised. His current GCS is E4, V4, M1. His observations are: BP 102/76, HR 112, RR 26, sats 93% on 4L with a temperature of 37.0°C. The trauma team are performing a primary and secondary survey.

a List five features indicative of spinal cord injury which would be seen in a spinal cord trauma patient during initial assessment. (5 marks)

i. ....

ii. ....

iii. ....

iv. ....

v. ....

b You are concerned that the patient's respiratory function is deteriorating. State three possible reasons for a potential difficult airway attributable to a trauma patient with suspected spinal cord injury. (3 marks)

i. ....

ii. ....

iii. ....

c Which respiratory muscles are affected by a spinal cord injury at the level indicated? Complete the table below. (3 marks)

Level of injury	Respiratory muscles affected (list one group)
Above C3	
Below C5 but above T8	
Below T8 but above L1	

You have successfully intubated the patient and commenced invasive ventilation. Fluid resuscitation and vasopressor treatment has commenced. The neurosurgical registrar at the accepting tertiary centre has accepted the patient for immediate transfer for fixation and due to concerns about the development of 'secondary cord injury'.

d   List two causes of secondary cord injury.   (2 marks)

i. ....

ii. ....

Two years later, the patient is admitted for debridement and washout of a sacral pressure sore. Since his spinal cord injury, he has had a long-term suprapubic catheter inserted under sedation, but has not had a general anaesthetic.

e   List three symptoms/signs of autonomic dysreflexia.   (3 marks)

i. ....

ii. ....

iii. ....

f   State two methods of managing autonomic dysreflexia, should it occur.   (2 marks)

i. ....

ii. ....

g   List two adverse sequelae of autonomic dysreflexia, if not treated urgently.   (2 marks)

i. ....

ii. ....

CRQ 3: Amniotic fluid embolism

A 36-year-old woman (G3P2) with no comorbidities is being induced for labour with an oxytocin infusion. She had an epidural inserted an hour previously which was reported to be working well. She has been nil by mouth and received no other medication. You have been asked to review her as she is now hypotensive, confused, breathless and has a headache. The midwife is also concerned about changes to the CTG trace baseline.

---

a List four obstetric and four non-obstetric differential diagnoses for her current condition. (4 marks)

Obstetric

i. ....

ii. ....

iii. ....

iv. ....

Non-obstetric

i. ....

ii. ....

iii. ....

iv. ....

Five minutes later, she has established cardiovascular collapse and advanced life support is commenced.

b What are the key differences between obstetric ALS and general adult ALS? (3 marks)

i. ....

ii. ....

iii. ....

c List and explain the two theories for the pathophysiology behind
the development of an amniotic fluid embolism. (6 marks)

i. Theory..

Explanation ....

....

ii. Theory...

Explanation ....

....

d List five surgical management strategies to control uterine atony. (5 marks)

i. ....

ii. ....

iii. ....

iv. ....

v. ....

e List two pharmacological agents with doses (other than blood products)
that are utilised in major obstetric haemorrhage to address coagulopathy
specifically. (2 marks)

i. ....

ii. ....

CRQ 4: Pulmonary hypertension

You review a 42-year-old man with a subacute history of worsening shortness of breath, marked pitting oedema and episodes of feeling faint. He is currently in atrial fibrillation with a fast ventricular rate of 136, but denies any chest pain. He has a past medical history of asthma, obesity, and has a hiatus hernia. He has a family history of pulmonary hypertension. An urgent echocardiogram is performed which suggests a pulmonary artery systolic pressure (PASP) of 45–55mmHg, along with a markedly dilated left atrium, right atrium and right ventricle.

a What grade of pulmonary hypertension is indicated by this patient's PASP? (1 mark)

....

b List any three of the five WHO classifications of pulmonary hypertension, and provide an example of each. (3 marks)

i. ....

ii. ....

iii. ....

c Complete the table below regarding pharmaco-therapeutic agents for arterial pulmonary hypertension. (5 marks)

Class of agent	Example drug(s) – list one if box empty
Prostanoids	
	bosentan, ambrisentan, macitentan
Nitric oxide pathway	
Inodilators	
Inotropes	

d You are due to assist a consultant with providing sedation to cardiovert this patient. What general physiological strategies are required to minimise rises in pulmonary hypertension and avoid deterioration? (4 marks)

....

....

....

....

e Pulmonary artery pressures can be reduced by attenuating hypoxic pulmonary vasoconstriction (HPV). List three determinants of HPV. (3 marks)

i. ....

ii. ....

iii. ....

f From the image below, for each section (A to D) indicate the location of the distal tip of pulmonary artery catheter AND the corresponding pressure range in mmHg. (4 marks)

Length of catheter advanced

A. ....

B. ....

C. ....

D. ....

CRQ 5: Chronic post-surgical pain

You are reviewing a 29-year-old man who has been finding it difficult to manage his pain 6 months after a dental extraction procedure.

---

a List three surgeries that have a >50% risk of resulting in chronic post-surgical pain (CPSP). (3 marks)

i. ....

ii. ....

iii. ....

b List five patient-related risk factors for developing CPSP. (5 marks)

i. ....

ii. ....

iii. ....

iv. ....

v. ....

c Define the following: (2 marks)

i. **Allodynia** ....

ii. **Hyperalgesia** ....

d State four regional anaesthetic techniques which may have some use in peri-operative analgesia for patients undergoing a mastectomy. (4 marks)

i. ....

ii. ....

iii. ....

iv. ....

e Complete the table below for the following analgesic agents. (4 marks)

Analgesic agent	Principal receptor/channel it acts on	Effect at receptor/channel
Parecoxib		
Clonidine		
Ketamine		
Gabapentin		

f Afferent neurones transmitting pain travel within which tracts in the spinal cord? (1 mark)

....

g List three cortical areas involved in the 'processing' of nociceptive signals. (3 marks)

i. ....

ii. ....

iii. ....

CRQ 6: Neonatal resus

You review a 3-day-old neonate in A&E suspected to have sepsis. The child was a normal vaginal delivery at 41 weeks and has Down's syndrome. At present, the child has been commenced on IV fluids and IV broad-spectrum antibiotics. The actual weight of the child is 4.0kg. You are called because the paediatric team are concerned that the patient is continuing to deteriorate.

a What are the most common infective organisms for sepsis in the newborn? (3 marks)

i. ....

ii. ....

iii. ....

b Calculate the appropriate **uncuffed** oral endotracheal tube size and length for this patient. (2 marks)

Tube size: ....

Tube length: ....

c Complete the table below with the correct doses for the drugs that may be required for this patient. (5 marks)

Medication	Correct dose for this patient (intravenous)
Atropine	
Adrenaline	
Suxamethonium	
Ketamine	
Cefuroxime	

d Outline how intravenous fluids will be used in circulatory shock in this patient. (3 marks)

....

....

....

e In the event of a cardiac arrest, describe the conduct of resuscitation for the sub-headings below. (3 marks)

CPR ratio: ....

Anatomical position of defibrillator pads: ....

Defibrillation energy: ....

f List four potential causes of a difficult airway in this patient. (4 marks)

i. ....

ii. ....

iii. ....

iv. ....

CRQ 7:   Statistics

You have been asked by a consultant colleague to prepare a presentation for your department's journal club. You have selected a number of articles and have been reviewing them to determine which would be most suitable.

a When would a researcher choose a retrospective study rather than a prospective study? (1 mark)

....

b List two disadvantages of using a retrospective study. (2 marks)

i. ....

ii. ....

c What is involved in each of the phases of a clinical trial, with regard to new drugs entering the market? (4 marks)

Phase 1: ....

Phase 2: ....

Phase 3: ....

Phase 4: ....

d Name the three main types of bias that may exist in a clinical trial. (3 marks)

i. ....

ii. ....

iii. ....

e Explain the following terms. (2 marks)

Type I error: ....

Type II error: ....

f   Explain the following terms.   (3 marks)

Sensitivity:..

Specificity: ....

Positive predictive value: ....

g   Rank the levels of scientific evidence by number.   (4 marks)

1. ....

2. ....

3. ....

4. ....

h   What is meant by the term 'meta-analysis'?   (1 mark)

....

CRQ 8: Anaphylaxis

A patient has been induced for an elective right hemi-colectomy for colon cancer. Aside from the cancer, she is 70kg and has only mild and usually well-controlled hypertension. She takes amlodipine 5mg once a day. She has had a previous laparoscopic cholecystectomy without any issue. She was given an induction with fentanyl, propofol, rocuronium and co-amoxiclav for surgical prophylaxis. 2 minutes later she becomes hypotensive (unrecordable NIBP) and tachycardic (HR 150). There is a sudden drop in etCO$_2$ to 1.2kPa and a drop in O$_2$ saturation to 70 on plethysmograph. You suspect the patient is suffering from anaphylaxis.

a According to NAP6, what is the incidence of peri-operative anaphylaxis? (1 mark)

....

b What are the most common causative agents of peri-operative anaphylaxis? (4 marks)

i. ....

ii. ....

iii. ....

iv. ....

c What is the mechanism underpinning the anaphylactoid/anaphylaxis reaction? (3 marks)

....

....

....

d Aside from hypotension, tachycardia, desaturation and decrease in etCO$_2$, list three other clinical features that may be present in an anaphylaxis reaction. (3 marks)

i. ....

ii. ....

iii. ....

e What is the immediate management of patients who are experiencing an anaphylactic reaction, including doses of treatment agents? (6 marks)

....

....

....

....

....

....

f What is the rate of adrenaline infusion that should be started if an anaphylaxis reaction is ongoing? (1 mark)

....

g What blood test should be taken for follow-up (1 mark), and over what timescales (1 mark) should it be taken?

i. ....

ii. Timescales ....

CRQ 9: Abdominal aortic aneurysm

The vascular registrar on call has informed the on-call theatre team that they are expecting a patient with a suspected ruptured abdominal aortic aneurysm (AAA) from another local hospital that they may wish to repair surgically as an emergency.

a What is the underlying pathophysiology underpinning the development of an AAA? (2 marks)

....

....

b List four risk factors that may lead to the development of an AAA. (4 marks)

i. ....

ii. ....

iii. ....

iv. ....

c In the elective setting, at what size of aneurysm should a patient be referred for consideration of surgery or an urgent vascular surgeon opinion? (1 mark)

....

The patient presents to the A&E department and the surgical and anaesthetic team have been asked to review the patient prior to theatre. He is hypotensive and tachycardic and on examination has a pulsatile abdominal mass.

d List three differentials other than a ruptured AAA for the patient's presentation. (3 marks)

i. ....

ii. ....

iii. ....

e Choose a scoring system for determining mortality in a AAA and list two of the variables used within it. (3 marks)

Scoring system: ....

i. Variable: ....

ii. Variable: ....

f List two complications of over-aggressive resuscitation with IV fluids to maintain a blood pressure prior to arriving in theatre. (2 marks)

i. ....

ii. ....

The patient is brought to theatre and has a successful 'opiate-heavy' induction with fentanyl, propofol and rocuronium. The surgery progresses quickly and the surgeon informs the theatre that they are about to cross-clamp the aorta.

g Describe the physiological response to aortic cross-clamping. (2 marks)

....

....

The surgery is completed and the patient is transferred to the intensive care unit for post-operative care. The operating surgeon is concerned about the possibility of abdominal compartment syndrome.

h At what value of pressure would abdominal compartment syndrome be considered? List two features that would make it more likely to develop post-operatively. (3 marks)

Value of pressure: ....

i. ....

ii. ....

CRQ 10:   Rhinological surgery

A 46-year-old female patient has presented for pre-assessment before undergoing functional endoscopic sinus surgery (FESS).

a List four patient or surgical factors that would make this patient unsuitable for day surgery. (4 marks)

i. ....

ii. ....

iii. ....

iv. ....

At pre-assessment the patient is found to have an ASA score of 1 and no other contraindications to day case procedures. The patient has been admitted for her FESS procedure. During the team brief the surgeons want to discuss anaesthetic options for minimising blood loss.

b What non-pharmacological measures can be used to limit blood loss in this case? (2 marks)

i. ....

ii. ....

c List three untoward effects which are more common when using cocaine, compared to other topical local anaesthetic and vasoconstrictor agents. (3 marks)

i. ....

ii. ....

iii. ....

d Explain what is meant by the term 'hypotensive anaesthesia'. (2 marks)

....

....

e List five patient factors or surgical reasons why a cuffed endotracheal tube rather than a supra-glottic airway might be used for this procedure. (5 marks)

i. ....

ii. ....

iii. ....

iv. ....

v. ....

The surgeon asks for a throat pack to be placed prior to the procedure.

f Describe four measures that can be used to reduce the risk of accidental retention of the throat pack. (4 marks)

i. ....

ii. ....

iii. ....

iv. ....

CRQ 11: Obstructive sleep apnoea

A 47-year-old man is listed for a sub-acromial decompression and shoulder arthroscopy. He is 156cm tall and weighs 128kg. He has concurrent hypertension, type 2 diabetes mellitus and familial hypercholesterolaemia. He is allergic to penicillin, and currently takes ramipril, metformin and atorvastatin. He is an ex-smoker, and consumes 14 units of alcohol a week. He describes his exercise tolerance as unrestricted and works as a warehouse supervisor. He has been researching online about his tiredness and he thinks he may be suffering from obstructive sleep apnoea (OSA).

---

a List six predisposing factors for OSA. (6 marks)

i. ....

ii. ....

iii. ....

iv. ....

v. ....

vi. ....

b What is the pathophysiology of OSA? (2 marks)

....

....

c List two methods used in the diagnosis of OSA. (2 marks)

i. ....

ii. ....

d   Complete the table below.   (3 marks)

Severity of OSA	Apnoea–hypopnoea Index (AHI) score
Mild	
Moderate	
Severe	

An ABG performed demonstrates a pCO_2 of 8.2kPa. You plan to postpone the surgery until the patient has undergone supervised weight loss and is established on continuous positive airway pressure (CPAP).

e   List four of the benefits of long-term CPAP therapy in OSA.   (4 marks)

i.   ....

ii.   ....

iii.   ....

iv.   ....

f   List three strategies to avoid enhanced post-operative pharyngeal muscle relaxation related to anaesthetic conduct.   (3 marks)

i.   ....

ii.   ....

iii.   ....

CRQ 12: Lung transplant

A 54-year-old man has been listed for an elective lung transplant. He is an ex-smoker and has a history of ischaemic heart disease. He has been getting progressively more short of breath over the last year and has been seen by the cardiothoracic surgeons, who have listed him for surgery.

a Name two conditions that may lead to a patient requiring a lung transplant. (2 marks)

i. ....

ii. ....

b What physiological, pathological or patient characteristics would mean that a patient can be considered for transplantation? (2 marks)

....

....

c Name four absolute contraindications to a patient having a lung transplant. (4 marks)

i. ....

ii. ....

iii. ....

iv. ....

d List four investigations you may order when seeing the patient in pre-assessment clinic, and give your rationale for why you would order them (excluding blood tests). (4 marks)

i. ....

ii. ....

iii. ....

iv. ....

e In which circumstances would it be appropriate to perform the surgery 'on-pump' rather than 'off-pump'? (2 marks)

i. ....

ii. ....

The operation proceeds uneventfully and the patient is transferred to the ICU post-operatively for post-transplantation care. The surgical team and anaesthetic team are worried about the potential for primary graft dysfunction post-operatively.

f After what length of transplant ischaemia time would you be concerned about the elevated risk of primary graft dysfunction? (1 mark)

....

g Patients with which underlying condition are more likely to develop primary graft dysfunction? (1 mark)

....

h What are the possible signs of primary graft dysfunction? (2 marks)

i. ....

ii. ....

i What is the usual regimen for post-operative immunosuppression? (2 marks)

....

....

SBA 1:

You have sited an epidural for labour in the maternity suite for a 23-year-old woman.

Which of the following is the last to be obtunded by local anaesthetics?

A. Sympathetic tone
B. Motor function
C. Sensation of cold
D. Proprioception
E. Sensation of touch

SBA 2:

A patient with severe Raynaud's phenomenon has been referred to the pain clinic for a stellate ganglion block to treat their symptoms.

Which of the following is not a complication of a stellate ganglion block?

A. Pneumothorax
B. Intercostal neuralgia
C. Mediastinitis
D. Mueller's syndrome
E. Perforated oesophagus

SBA 3:

A 58-year-old woman has presented for partial lobectomy for lung cancer, which will require one-lung ventilation. She has severe rheumatoid arthritis with atlanto-axial subluxation and temporomandibular joint dysfunction. Upon airway assessment, her inter-incisor distance is less than 2 finger breadths.

What would be the most appropriate intubation technique and endotracheal tube for this procedure?

A. AFOI and Robertshaw double-lumen tube
B. AFOI and bronchial blocker
C. AFOI and endobronchial intubation
D. Videolaryngoscopy and Robertshaw double-lumen tube
E. Videolaryngoscopy and bronchial blocker

SBA 4:

A 54-year-old woman presents to A&E with a severe headache, neck stiffness and double vision. Her symptoms have been ongoing for several weeks, but have been gradually worsening over the last day. She also complains of feeling extremely nauseous and has vomited four times since the headaches began to worsen. She has a family history of polycystic kidney disease, but is otherwise fit and well.

What is the gold standard choice of investigation for this patient?

A. Digital subtraction angiography (DSA) of the brain
B. CT head with contrast
C. MRA (magnetic resonance angiography) of the brain
D. CT venogram of the brain
E. MRI brain

SBA 5:

A 26-year-old G1P0 woman has an epidural *in situ* for labour analgesia. The midwives are concerned, as the patient still appears to be in some pain and despite 1cm withdrawal of the epidural catheter and single bolus of local anaesthetic, it still does not appear to be effective. According to the epidural notes it was difficult to site, with multiple attempts at different levels. After removing the catheter and attempting to re-site it, the patient has an inadvertent dural puncture during the procedure.

What is the most appropriate way to manage this dural puncture and the patient's pain relief?

A. Remove the needle and re-attempt at the space above
B. Thread the catheter and use it as an intrathecal catheter
C. Remove the needle and offer the patient a remifentanil infusion
D. Remove the needle and offer the patient a morphine PCA
E. Perform a low dose CSE

SBA 6:

Which of the following is true regarding the anatomy of the trachea?

A. There are 8 bronchopulmonary segments in the right lung
B. The trachea is composed of 8–10 C-shaped cartilaginous rings
C. The trachealis muscle forms the posterior wall of the trachea
D. The trachea terminates at level T5/T6 in the supine patient
E. The lingular segments occur in the right lung

SBA 7:

A 68-year-old woman with a long history of smoking has been listed for laser debulking of a laryngeal tumour.

From the list below, select the most appropriate lasing medium for this surgery.

A. Ruby (red 694nm)
B. Argon (blue green 500nm)
C. CO_2 (far infrared 10600nm)
D. Holmium:YAG (mid infrared 2070nm)
E. Nd:YAG (near infrared 1064nm)

SBA 8:

A 51-year-old man is brought to A&E after sustaining severe burns from a house fire. The burns cover his face, chest, stomach and both arms. He is approximately 80kg.

What is the approximate volume of fluid replacement required over 24 hours?

A. 10560ml
B. 7680ml
C. 8640ml
D. 14400ml
E. 12960ml

SBA 9:

A 72-year-old woman with a background of multiple sclerosis is referred to the pain clinic with a new headache and associated facial pain. The pain is electric shock-like in nature, intermittent and has no obvious trigger. She has no neurological deficit.

What is the first-line treatment for this condition?

A. Amitriptyline
B. Facial nerve blockade
C. Gabapentin
D. Carbamazepine
E. Surgical decompression

SBA 10:

A 39-year-old woman is booked for an elective caesarean section after pre-natal screening of the foetus noted transposition of the great arteries (TGA).

What will be the immediate management of this neonate after delivery?

A. Balloon atrial septostomy
B. Immediate surgical repair
C. Start prostaglandin infusion
D. Start nitrate infusion
E. Immediate intubation and ventilation

SBA 11:

A 62-year-old woman is having a pleural tap in the ICU for a large effusion. A sample is sent to the pathology laboratory and results are as follows:
- LDH 1400IU/L
- Glucose 1.0mmol/L
- pH 7.1
- Amylase 20

What is the next best investigation or management of this patient's pleural effusion?

A. Interventional radiology-guided chest drain
B. CT staging scan
C. IV diuretics
D. Referral to thoracic surgeons
E. Seldinger chest drain

SBA 12:

Midway through a laparoscopic right hemi-colectomy on a normally fit and well 53-year-old man, the three-lead ECG on the anaesthetic monitor shows significant ST elevation.

What is the most appropriate first step in the management of this patient?

A. Stop the surgery
B. Administer 100% oxygen
C. Commence an IV glyceryl trinitrate infusion
D. Obtain an urgent 12-lead ECG
E. Deepen the plane of anaesthesia

SBA 13:

A 48-year-old man with chronic kidney disease stage 4 is administered sodium bicarbonate prior to emergency surgery on the renal ward. Upon review, the patient's arm is swollen around the site of the cannula and he is complaining of severe arm pain.

Which of the following is not a recommended treatment strategy for extravasation?

A. Saline washout
B. Liposuction
C. Hydrocortisone
D. Hyaluronidase
E. Cold compress

SBA 14:

According to the MBRRACE-UK: *Saving Lives, Improving Mothers' Care* report (2020), what is the most common cause of maternal death during pregnancy or in the first 6 weeks post-partum in the UK?

A. Venous thromboembolism
B. Maternal mental health issues and suicide
C. Cardiac disease
D. Eclampsia
E. Bleeding

SBA 15:

You are about to anaesthetise an 8-year-old boy who is undergoing correctional surgery for his idiopathic scoliosis.

Which of the following anaesthetic agents is least likely to alter the sensory and/or motor evoked potentials, during electrophysiological monitoring?

A. Sevoflurane
B. Midazolam
C. Ketamine
D. Morphine
E. Nitrous oxide

SBA 16:

A 74-year-old woman is due to undergo a video-assisted thoracotomy (VATS) and pneumonectomy for lung cancer. She is concerned about pain relief after the operation, as she has chronic neuropathic pain following a left-sided mastectomy 20 years ago.

Which option would be the ideal technique for pain management?

A. Thoracic epidural
B. Paravertebral block
C. Intrathecal opiate
D. Post-op patient-controlled analgesia (PCA)
E. Intercostal blocks

SBA 17:

A 67-year-old man is due to undergo an elective left knee arthroscopy as a day case. He weighs 71kg.

Which of the following neuraxial local anaesthetics and dose is most appropriate to allow the patient to be discharged on the same day, and be sufficient for the operative time?

A. Bupivacaine 0.1mg/kg
B. Prilocaine 40mg
C. Ropivacaine 0.1mg/kg
D. Prilocaine 60mg
E. Lidocaine 10mg

SBA 18:

A patient in the post-operative care unit has been complaining of worsening chest pain and shortness of breath. The recovery nurses have performed an ECG which demonstrates ST elevation in leads II and III, and aVF and ST depression in aVL.

Which coronary artery is most likely to be the cause of these ECG changes?

A. Left anterior descending
B. Left circumflex
C. Right coronary artery
D. Left main stem
E. Left marginal

SBA 19:

A 32-year-old man presents for an emergency laparoscopic cholecystectomy. He has a history of an obstructive tracheal tumour which was treated 5 years ago. He is regularly followed up for this, and is currently asymptomatic with no obvious recurrence.

Which of the following treatment modalities for tracheal tumours that this patient may have undergone would require **mandatory** use of fibre-optic intubation for surgery in this instance?

A. Argon plasma coagulation
B. Forceps debulking
C. Brachytherapy
D. Cryotherapy
E. Tracheobronchial stenting

SBA 20:

A 92-year-old patient is scheduled for an elective cataract removal to be performed under local anaesthesia. The patient has a mechanical heart valve and has been on warfarin since their valve replacement, with an INR target of 2.5–3.5. They are also on 75mg of aspirin once daily.

Which of the following options best describes the management of their peri-operative anticoagulation?

A. The patient should continue warfarin with no change to target INR
B. The patient should stop warfarin and be bridged with low molecular weight heparin
C. The patient should continue warfarin and receive tranexamic acid pre-operatively
D. The patient should stop warfarin 7 days pre-operatively, then re-start when the operation is complete
E. The operation should be performed under general anaesthesia

SBA 21:

A 16-year-old girl presents to the pain clinic with severe pain in her left leg. The pain is burning in nature and not relieved by over-the-counter medication. She reports that touch, including wearing trousers, exacerbates the pain. She has a provisional diagnosis of complex regional pain syndrome (CRPS).

Which of the following is not part of the Budapest criteria for CRPS?

A. Weakness in affected limb
B. Muscle atrophy in affected limb
C. Skin colour changes in affected limb
D. Swelling of affected limb
E. Changes to hair distribution in affected limb

SBA 22:

A 3-year-old child, who is known to have a congenital genetic disorder, presents for tonsillectomy.

Which of the following congenital disorders has the greatest risk of causing difficult bag-mask ventilation in a child?

A. Apert syndrome
B. Treacher Collins syndrome
C. Pierre Robin sequence
D. Cleft lip and palate
E. Gaucher disease

SBA 23:

Which is the correct daily basal nutritional requirement for a patient with critical illness in the intensive care unit?

A. 50ml/kg water
B. 1–2mmol/kg calcium
C. 1g/kg fat
D. 0.8–1.2mmol/kg magnesium
E. 5g/kg carbohydrate

SBA 24:

A 48-year-old man with end-stage liver disease presents to A&E acutely anaemic following five large episodes of haematemesis. The massive transfusion protocol is activated and the patient receives 5 units of packed red blood cells, 5 units of FFP and 2 units of platelets. Following this the patient becomes hypotensive with a narrow pulse pressure. The patient's ECG shows a prolonged QT interval and flattened ST segments.

What immediate management is required?

A. Rapid rewarming with forced air warmer
B. IV insulin and dextrose
C. IV sodium bicarbonate
D. 500ml bolus of IV fluid
E. IV calcium gluconate

SBA 25:

Which of the opioid receptor subtypes is most responsible for causing respiratory depression?

A. Mu
B. Kappa
C. Delta
D. Nociceptin
E. Gamma

SBA 26:

You review a 37-week pregnant, 22-year-old woman (G2P1) for maternal hypotension (84/48mmHg) which has been refractory to IV fluids. The cause is suspected to be sepsis, and a plan has been made to deliver the foetus once haemodynamic stability is established. She has been transferred to theatre for rapid stabilisation.

Which of the following is the most appropriate vasopressor to commence?

A. Adrenaline
B. Ephedrine
C. Arginine vasopressin
D. Noradrenaline
E. Dobutamine

SBA 27:

A 45-year-old woman has sustained a head injury after tripping and hitting her head on a low wall. The ambulance crew state that witnesses at the scene described her as conscious immediately after the injury, and she remains conscious in A&E. She has had two episodes of vomiting in the ambulance. On your initial assessment, she is confused but obeying simple motor commands and her eyes open spontaneously. There is a 4cm wound on her head in the left fronto-temporal region.

Which of the following factors would suggest she requires CT imaging of her head?

A. Glasgow Coma Score (GCS) of 14 on initial assessment in the ED
B. Mechanism of injury
C. Age
D. Vomiting twice since injury
E. Presence of head wound

SBA 28:

A 62-year-old man presents for a transurethral resection of the prostate (TURP). He has had one previous TIA and on review of his pre-operative ECG he has pathological Q waves. He also has a history of hypertension and type 2 diabetes on metformin.

When calculating his risk using Lee's revised cardiac index (2017 update), what is his likelihood of having a peri-operative cardiovascular complication?

A. 0.3%
B. 2.4%
C. 3.9%
D. 10.1%
E. 15.6%

SBA 29:

Your colleague comes to see you in a state of distress, as they have just performed a wrong-sided block for a patient on their operating list.

The following are thought to increase risk of wrong-sided block except for:

A. Mark or sticker placed by anaesthetic practitioner
B. >1 block performed
C. Patient repositioning
D. Use of mild sedation
E. Inadequate information from the patient

SBA 30:

A 70-year-old woman is undergoing an emergency laparotomy for a small bowel obstruction. An oesophageal Doppler is being used for cardiac output monitoring.

Which of the following parameters most accurately indicates the preload of the left ventricle?

A. Corrected flow time (FTc)
B. Peak velocity (PV)
C. Cycle time (CT)
D. Mean acceleration
E. Minute distance

SBA 31:

When topicalising the airway in preparation for awake fibre-optic intubation, which of the following is the most appropriate maximum dose of local anaesthetic?

A. Lidocaine 5mg/kg without adrenaline
B. Lidocaine 7mg/kg with adrenaline
C. Prilocaine 6mg/kg without adrenaline
D. Cocaine 3mg/kg
E. Lidocaine 9mg/kg without adrenaline

SBA 32:

A 78-year-old woman has presented for vitreoretinal surgery. She has a medical history of atrial fibrillation (on edoxaban) and well-controlled Parkinson's. She undergoes a successful peribulbar block and has been recovering in the post-operative recovery room. She develops a sudden onset proptosis with headache and reduced visual acuity.

What is the most likely cause of her symptoms?

A. Ecchymosis
B. Retro-bulbar haemorrhage
C. Globe injury
D. Muscular palsy
E. Optic nerve atrophy

SBA 33:

As part of the acute pain ward round, you review a 32-year-old man who has been using a morphine PCA (1mg bolus/5 minutes). He had undergone a reconstructive procedure of his left forearm, and a regional nerve catheter was avoided due to a presumed high risk of compartment syndrome. In the last 24 hours, he had required 60mg of morphine via the PCA.

Choose the correct conversion to oral medication from the list below.

A. 60mg of modified release oral morphine – BD regularly, and 30mg of immediate release oral morphine 6-hourly PRN
B. 120mg of modified release oral morphine – BD regularly, and 30mg of immediate release oral morphine 4-hourly PRN
C. 90mg of modified release oral morphine – BD regularly, and 20mg of immediate release oral morphine 4-hourly PRN
D. 60mg of modified release oral morphine – BD regularly, and 10mg of immediate release oral morphine 4-hourly PRN
E. 90mg of modified release oral morphine – BD regularly, and 10mg of immediate release oral morphine 4-hourly PRN

SBA 34:

A 5-year-old boy is awaiting bowel surgery for a possible bowel carcinoma. He has been prescribed bowel prep as part of the pre-surgery work-up.

With regard to starvation time, how long prior to the operation should bowel prep be consumed?

A. 2 hours
B. 4 hours
C. 6 hours
D. 8 hours
E. 10 hours

SBA 35:

A 59-year-old man has been admitted to the ICU following an episode of reduced consciousness at home. His past medical history is unclear, but he has had a CT head/chest/abdomen/pelvis which is suspicious for lung malignancy with liver and bone metastases. He has been found to have a serum corrected calcium of 3.4g/dl.

What is the most likely ECG abnormality that would be seen in this patient?

A. Widening of the QRS complex
B. Prolonged QTc
C. Delta waves
D. Shortened QTc
E. Narrowing of the QRS complex

SBA 36:

A 72-year-old patient presents to the anaesthetic pre-operative assessment clinic as he is due to undergo a transurethral resection of the prostate (TURP). On the rhythm strip of his ECG there is a marginally widened QRS complex and intermittently non-conducted p waves. The non-conducted waves happen regularly after every third complex. He is asymptomatic and his exercise tolerance is normal.

What is the correct pre-operative intervention/investigation for this patient?

A. Permanent pacemaker insertion
B. No intervention required
C. Pre-operative angiogram
D. Echocardiogram
E. CPEX testing

SBA 37:

A 78-year-old man with severe Parkinson's disease presents to the pre-operative assessment clinic prior to an elective knee arthroscopy.

Which of the following medications' mechanism of action is to prevent breakdown of dopamine by catechol-O-methyltransferase (COMT) inhibition?

A. Apomorphine
B. Rotigotine
C. Pramipexole
D. Tolcapone
E. Selegiline

SBA 38:

You are fast-bleeped to review a 43-year-old woman in the delivery suite (G1P0, 40+2), who had an induction of labour for advanced maternal age. The obstetrician is concerned about foetal distress as per the CTG and uterine hyperactivity, and would like to take the patient to theatre for a category 2 emergency caesarean section.

What would be the next appropriate step?

A. Give oxygen – 15L via NRBM
B. Terbutaline 5mcg IV
C. 250ml of Hartmann's fluid IV
D. Stop oxytocin infusion
E. Magnesium 1.2g IV

SBA 39:

A 24-year-old man attends the neurosurgical unit for an elective craniotomy for a large glioma. The neurosurgeons wish to perform this awake with neurofunctional mapping during the dissection phase. He has no other comorbidities and has not had any previous surgeries.

What would be the ideal induction peri-operative strategy for this patient?

A. Sedation with midazolam and scalp block by surgeons
B. Induction with propofol, remifentanil and rocuronium and endotracheal intubation
C. Induction with propofol and remifentanil and endotracheal intubation
D. Induction with propofol, remifentanil and rocuronium and insertion of supraglottic airway
E. Induction with propofol and remifentanil and insertion of supraglottic airway

SBA 40:

Which of the following conditions would not be an indication for cardiac transplantation?

A. Advanced heart failure with New York Heart Association class III or IV functional status with recurrent hospitalisations despite maximal medical therapy

B. Recurrent life-threatening ventricular arrhythmias despite an implantable cardiac defibrillator (ICD)

C. Acute cardiogenic shock, requiring infusions of inotropic agents or temporary mechanical circulatory support

D. Refractory angina without further therapeutic options

E. Severe left ventricular dysfunction with severe cardio-hepatic liver dysfunction

SBA 41:

Which of the following regional anaesthetic techniques has the highest risk of haemorrhagic complications in patients with abnormal coagulation?

A. Interscalene brachial plexus block

B. Axillary brachial plexus block

C. Stellate ganglion block

D. Intercostal nerve block

E. Epidural with catheter

SBA 42:

A patient has been anaesthetised for an emergency laparotomy.

With regard to heat loss during an operation, which of the following contributes to the highest percentage?

A. Conduction

B. Convection

C. Evaporation

D. Respiration

E. Radiation

SBA 43:

A 31-year-old woman presents for a total thyroidectomy. You decide to place a NIM tube.

What does NIM stand for?

A. Neuronal injury monitor
B. Neural integrity monitor
C. Negative integrity modulator
D. Neural induction monitor
E. Neuronal induction modulator

SBA 44:

A 70-year-old man has presented for a carotid endarterectomy following a transient ischaemic attack (TIA) one week ago. He has been found to have an 80% stenosis of his right internal carotid artery. Three weeks ago, he was admitted to hospital following an MI and had three drug-eluting cardiac stents inserted. He has since been on both aspirin and clopidogrel.

What is the safest way to manage this patient's antiplatelet agents in the peri-operative phase?

A. Pause surgery until at least 3 months following stent placement
B. Continue with the surgery on aspirin and clopidogrel
C. Continue with the surgery on aspirin only, temporarily hold clopidogrel
D. Switch the aspirin and clopidogrel to treatment-dose LMWH
E. Switch the aspirin and clopidogrel to IV heparin infusion

SBA 45:

Which of the following tests is not routinely used to determine whether back pain is emanating from the sacroiliac joint?

A. Compression test (approximation test)
B. Patrick's sign (flexion abduction external rotation test)
C. Thigh thrust test (posterior shear test)
D. Fortin's finger test
E. Keogh's manoeuvre

SBA 46:

A 5-year-old, 18kg boy has presented to the day surgery unit for a circumcision. After discussing the anaesthetic options, the patient's mother has consented for a combination of general anaesthesia and caudal block.

What is the appropriate volume of local anaesthetic (bupivacaine 0.25%) to be used for the caudal block?

A. 9ml
B. 18ml
C. 20ml
D. 22ml
E. 30ml

SBA 47:

A 65-year-old man is having a tracheostomy sited on ICU as part of a respiratory weaning strategy, having been on a ventilator for 7 days. After positioning the patient, giving muscle relaxant and sedation, the tracheostomy checklist is completed. After reviewing the checklist and cleaning the skin, the patient begins to become hypoxic with oxygen saturations of 86%.

What is the safest way to proceed?

A. Increase sedation and reassess
B. Reduce sedation and reassess
C. Bolus of IV adrenaline
D. Abandon the procedure
E. Continue with tracheostomy

SBA 48:

A 74-year-old man has been transferred to the intensive care unit following semi-elective surgery for an abdominal aortic aneurysm. He required a massive transfusion during the procedure, receiving 11 units of packed red cells. He has a past medical history of obesity (BMI 41) and hypertension. The surgery was successful and surgical closure was complete. Over 6 hours, his urine output has continued to decrease and he is now complaining of severe abdominal pain. He has also become hypercarbic (paCO$_2$ 8.6kPa) and hypotensive (88/39mmHg).

What is the most likely cause?

A. Surgical dehiscence
B. Hypovolaemia
C. Ventilator-associated pneumonia
D. Bowel injury during surgery
E. Abdominal compartment syndrome

SBA 49:

A 23-year-old woman has been brought into A&E by ambulance after being found collapsed in her parents' garage. She is noted to have a fluctuating conscious level and is incoherent. An ABG is taken and the results are as follows:

pH	7.13
pO_2	13.7kPa
pCO_2	2.6kPa
Lactate	4.7mmol/L
Na^+	140mmol/L
K^+	5.5mmol/L
Cl^-	108mmol/L
HCO_3^-	10mmol/L
Glucose	10.3mmol/L

What is the most appropriate treatment for this patient?

A. Insulin and dextrose infusion
B. Fixed rate insulin infusion
C. Ethanol
D. Sodium bicarbonate
E. Continuous veno-venous haemofiltration (CVVHF)

SBA 50:

You are due to anaesthetise a 26-year-old woman for an emergency appendicectomy. She is 16 weeks pregnant (G1P0), with no other medical or drug history of note.

Which of the following statements is false?

A. Open surgery is preferred to laparoscopy
B. Aortocaval compression must be accounted for from 13 weeks
C. Antacid prophylaxis is recommended after 14 weeks
D. Glycopyrrolate is safe in pregnancy
E. Neostigmine is unsafe in pregnancy

SBA 51:

A 55-year-old patient has been transferred to the neuro-critical care following a road traffic accident with a prolonged reduced GCS. A jugular bulb catheter has been inserted to measure jugular venous oxygen saturation.

Which of the following pathologies would result in a low sjVO$_2$?

A. Seizure
B. Cerebral infarction
C. Hypercapnia
D. Hypothermia
E. Vasodilation

SBA 52:

A 59-year-old man who underwent a mitral valve repair 3 hours previously is in cardiac arrest on the cardiac ICU. Resuscitation commences as per the modified cardiac-ALS protocol. He is noted to have an intra-aortic balloon pump (IABP) *in situ*.

What is the correct management of the IABP in this situation?

A. Turn off the IABP
B. Switch from a 2:1 to 1:1 ratio
C. Change to an ECG-based trigger
D. Remove the IABP
E. Change to a pressure-based trigger

SBA 53:

You are due to perform an ultrasound-guided femoral nerve block prior to an elective hip replacement.

Which of the following ultrasound probes, and their settings, is most appropriate for the ideal sonographic image?

A. Linear probe, 5–10MHz, 1–5cm depth
B. Linear probe, 2–5MHz, >5cm depth
C. Curvilinear probe, 2–5MHz, <5cm depth
D. Curvilinear probe, 5–10MHz, >5cm depth
E. Linear probe, 5–10MHz, 0.5–2cm depth

SBA 54:

What is the level of evidence achieved in a well-designed cohort study?

A. 1a
B. 1b
C. 2a
D. 2b
E. 3

SBA 55:

Which of the following congenital conditions is not known to cause any difficulty with airway management for the anaesthetist?

A. Morquio syndrome
B. Pierre Robin sequence
C. Apert syndrome
D. Goldenhar syndrome
E. Joubert syndrome

SBA 56:

A 45-year-old woman is to undergo a free-flap reconstruction of her breast following a mastectomy for breast cancer. The surgical team has opted to perform a DIEP flap. The patient is otherwise fit and well and has no other comorbidities.

What is the most important haemodynamic goal to optimise flap perfusion and operative success?

A. Maintain the haematocrit between 20% and 25%
B. Maintain the MAP >75mmHg with a phenylephrine infusion
C. IV fluids to maintain urine output at 1–2ml/kg/hr
D. Prevent hypothermia using warming devices
E. Therapeutic subcutaneous heparin

SBA 57:

Spinal cord stimulators (SCS) are used in adults with chronic neuropathic pain.

Which of the following is not an instance that requires an implanted SCS to be turned off?

A. Magnetic resonance imaging (MRI) scan
B. Pregnancy
C. Computed tomography (CT) scan
D. Cardiac defibrillation
E. Lithotripsy

SBA 58:

A 25-year-old man presents to the pre-operative assessment clinic before an elective cholecystectomy. The patient has an extensive surgical history due to congenital heart disease. The patient underwent several surgical interventions as a child and has been left with a Fontan (single ventricle) circulation.

Which of the following pre-operative investigations is not usually indicated for patients with a Fontan circulation?

A. Full blood count
B. Spirometry
C. Echocardiogram
D. 12-lead ECG
E. Renal function tests

SBA 59:

An 18-year-old woman presents to A&E after ingesting 45 tablets of paracetamol. She is drowsy, responsive only to pain, and has a systolic blood pressure of 74mmHg. After discussion with the local liver transplant unit, she is immediately transferred and placed on the liver transplant list.

Which of the following criteria does not form part of the King's College criteria for liver transplant?

A. Acidosis with pH <7.3 after resuscitation
B. Creatinine >300micromoles/L
C. Bilirubin >3mg/dl
D. Grade 3 encephalopathy
E. INR >6.5

SBA 60:

A 61-year-old man is in cardiac arrest on the general medical ward. CPR is ongoing and one dose of adrenaline and one dose of amiodarone have been administered to the patient, as well as three DC shocks. The patient was in VF initially, and at the next rhythm check was found to still be in VF.

What is the next step in pharmacological management for this patient in cardiac arrest?

A. Amiodarone
B. Adrenaline
C. Lidocaine
D. Magnesium
E. Flecainide

CRQ 1: answer guidance

Syllabus	NA_IK_02, N3_IK_21
Question type	Moderate: pass mark 12
Topic	**Brainstem death and brainstem death testing**
Aim	To understand the sequences required to confirm brainstem death and understand the underlying physiology of brainstem death.
Pass requirements	Understand how to confirm brainstem death and appropriately prepare a patient for donation.

Q	Answer	Marks	Guidance
a	• Deeply unconscious • Apnoeic • Mechanically ventilated • Known irreversible brain damage (or cause of brain damage)	1 1 1 1	Can accept variations on language used for unconscious.
b	**Pupillary response:** S = Optic (II) M = Oculomotor (III) Direct and consensual reflex sought by shining a bright light into each eye in turn **Oculo-vestibular reflex:** S = Vestibulocochlear (VIII) M = Oculomotor (III), trochlear (IV), abducens (VI) Injection of 50ml of ice-cold water into external auditory meatus **Response to pain:** S = Trigeminal (V) M = Facial (VII) Pain stimulus to supraorbital fissure	6	1 mark for correct pair of nerves. 1 mark for test.
c	• Vasopressin for diabetes insipidus • Methylprednisolone to increase extravascular lung water index • Thyroxine for functional hypothyroidism after hypothalamic ischaemia • Desmopressin for diabetes insipidus • Insulin for normoglycaemia	3	1 mark per correct pair.

Q	Answer	Marks	Guidance
d	• Reduced vasomotor tone due to loss of spinal cord sympathetic activity	1	
	• Reduced cardiac output due to vasodilation	1	
	• Reduced aortic diastolic pressure due to reduced preload and afterload	1	
	• Impaired myocardial perfusion due to reduced aortic diastolic pressure	1	
e	• Positive for: HIV, hep B/C, HTLV, syphilis, malaria	3	1 mark per correct answer.
	• Untreated systemic sepsis		Can also access previous patient refusal or lack of family consent.
	• Evidence of vCJD		
	• Progressive neurological disease: Alzheimer's/MND/Parkinson's		
	• Malignancy		
	• End organ damage from hypertension		
	• End organ damage from diabetes mellitus		
	• Previous transplant patient who has received immunosuppressive therapy		

There are a number of physiological changes that the brainstem-dead patient undergoes and it is important to be able to recognise these and treat these as soon as possible to allow for a smooth donation. This is obviously all guided by the patient's previous wishes or family wishes (despite current opt-out guidelines). There are a number of contraindications to donation but anyone suspected to be a potential donor should be discussed at the earliest opportunity with the receiving donation team, who will be able to offer advice.

Oram, J. and Murphy, P. (2011) Diagnosis of death. *CEACCP*, **11(3)**: 77–81.

Thomas, I. and Manara, A. (2020) Pitfalls in the diagnosis of death using neurological criteria. *BJA Education*, **20(1)**: 2–4.

CRQ 2: answer guidance

Syllabus	NA_IK_02, NA_IK_13, NA_IK_14
Question type	Hard: pass mark 10
Topic	**Spinal cord trauma and autonomic dysreflexia**
Aim	To correctly diagnose and stabilise a patient with a spinal cord injury as well as the management of autonomic dysreflexia.
Pass requirements	List the signs of spinal cord injury successfully.

Q	Answer	Marks	Guidance
a	• Hypotension • Bradycardia • Peripherally warm • Hypothermia • Flaccidity • Areflexia • Priapism • Loss/change in pain sensation below level of injury • Loss/change in touch sensation below level of injury • Loss/change in proprioception below level of injury • Loss/change in vibration sense below level of injury • Diaphragmatic breathing • Tachypnoea • Reduced vital capacity/PEFR	5	1 mark per correct answer. Should not accept 'neurogenic shock/spinal shock' as these are non-specific terms. Can accept respiratory failure.
b	• C-spine imobilisation • Physical presence of blocks/collar • Cricoid pressure may not be applied • May have concurrent max fax trauma • Contaminated airway (blood, vomit) • Airway oedema	3	1 mark per correct answer. Can also accept haemodynamic instability – although not specifically about airway, can also lead to difficulty in securing the airway.
c	Above C3: the diaphragm	1	Can also accept phrenic nerve for C3.
	Below C5 but above T8: inspiratory intercostal muscles (external)	1	
	Below T8 but above L1: expiratory intercostal muscles (internal) and abdominal muscles	1	
d	• Haemorrhage • Oedema • Hypoperfusion • Cord ischaemia	2	1 mark per correct answer.
e	• Unopposed hypertension • Headache • Nasal congestion • Facial flushing • Sweating • Pallor • Cool peripheries • Piloerection	3	1 mark per correct answer.

Q	Answer	Marks	Guidance
f	**Non-pharmacological:** • Sit patient upright • Loosen tight clothes • Empty bladder/catheterise/empty urinary catheter • Empty bowels/manual evacuation of faeces **Pharmacological:** • Sublingual/IV GTN • Sublingual nifedipine • IV hydralazine • IV diazoxide • Increase depth of anaesthesia • IV phentolamine • IV magnesium	2	1 mark per correct answer.
g	• Seizures • Intracerebral haemorrhage • Myocardial infarction • Pulmonary oedema • Bradyarrhythmias	2	1 mark per correct answer. Should not accept hypertension or 'arrhythmias' as these are too non-specific.

Acute spinal cord injury can be hard to diagnose on signs and symptoms alone and will often need imaging. These patients are usually trauma patients so may also have other coexisting pathologies which will need concurrent treatment. In an unstable C-spine fracture the gold standard management is surgical fixation, and it is important in the acute phase to prevent further secondary cord injury (much like avoiding secondary brain injury). Autonomic dysreflexia is a complication of a previous spinal cord injury which can cause swings in blood pressure and heart rate and can have severe complications. These patients should have invasive monitoring and high dependency care.

Bonner, S. and Smith, C. (2013) Initial management of acute spinal cord injury. *CEACCP*, **13(6)**: 224–231.

Petsas, A. and Drake, J. (2015) Perioperative management for patients with a chronic spinal cord injury. *BJA Education*, **15(3)**: 123–130.

CRQ 3: answer guidance

Syllabus	OB_IK_05
Question type	Moderate: pass mark 12
Topic	**Amniotic fluid embolism**
Aim	To be able to diagnose an amniotic fluid embolism and instigate the immediate management.
Pass requirements	Describe the pathophysiology of amniotic fluid embolism.

Q	Answer	Marks	Guidance
a	**Obstetric:** Eclampsia, uterine rupture, placental abruption, acute obstetric haemorrhage, peripartum cardiomyopathy, uterine inversion, amniotic fluid embolism **Non-obstetric:** Pulmonary embolism, air embolism, fat embolism, pulmonary oedema, pneumothorax, heart failure, myocardial infarction, anaphylaxis, sepsis, local anaesthetic toxicity, intracranial haemorrhage	4	1 mark per correct pair of answers.
b	• Neonatal and maternity arrest calls • Left-sided uterine displacement • Perimortem caesarean section within 4 minutes	1 1 1	The important thing to consider is the need for a neonatologist to attend as well as a maternity team.
c	**Mechanical theory** • Mechanical obstruction • by amniotic fluid and/or its components **Immune-mediated theory** • Anaphylactoid reaction secondary to amniotic fluid and/or its components • Activation of the coagulation cascade	1 1 1 1 1 1	Anaphylaxis should not be accepted as this is not necessarily true, but can accept mast cell degranulation.
d	• Intrauterine balloon tamponade • Bimanual uterine compression • Uterine compression sutures • Uterine artery embolisation • Pelvic vessel ligation • Intra-arterial balloon occlusion • Uterine packing • Hysterectomy	5	1 mark per correct answer.
e	Calcium chloride 10%, 10ml Tranexamic acid, 1g	1 1	Doses required to gain mark.

Amniotic fluid embolism is a rare but potentially fatal complication that can occur in pregnancy but also following birth. It has high mortality and the management is often supportive as there is no definitive treatment. The diagnosis is often made post mortem but having a high degree of suspicion will mean early haemodynamic management. Anyone who works on a labour ward should be familiar with the differences between traditional resus and resus in the obstetric population.

Dedhia, J. and Mushambi, M. (2007) Amniotic fluid embolism. *CEACCP*, **7(5):** 152–156.

Metodiev, Y., Ramasamy, P. and Tuffnel, D. (2018) Amniotic fluid embolism. *BJA Education*, **18:** 234–238.

CRQ 4: answer guidance

Syllabus	PR_IK_05, PB_IK_07
Question type	Hard: pass mark 10
Topic	**Pulmonary hypertension and hypoxic pulmonary vasoconstriction**
Aim	To recall the classes of pulmonary hypertension and anaesthetic considerations that govern hypoxic pulmonary vasoconstriction.
Pass requirements	Display an understanding of pulmonary hypertension and its relevant pharmacological and physiological management.

Q	Answer	Marks	Guidance
a	Moderate pulmonary hypertension	1	Can accept intermediate.
b	• Pulmonary artery hypertension *and one of:* Idiopathic/familial/portal hypertension/congenital heart disease/HIV/collagen vascular disease (e.g. scleroderma or lupus)/drugs/toxins • Pulmonary hypertension due to left heart disease *and one of:* Coronary heart disease/hypertension/myocardial damage (including MI)/valvular heart disease/age/systolic dysfunction/diastolic dysfunction • Lung disease *and one of:* COPD/interstitial lung disease/sleep apnoea/high altitude/alveolar hypoventilation • Chronic thromboembolic pulmonary hypertension *and one of:* Recurrent pulmonary emboli/large pulmonary embolus • Miscellaneous/unclear mechanisms *and one of:* Sarcoidosis/sickle cell anaemia/haemolytic anaemia/splenectomy/thyroid disease/Gaucher disease/vasculitis/glycogen storage disease/myeloproliferative disorders/neurofibromatosis	3	1 mark per correct answer. No half marks, so full example and description needed to gain mark.

Q	Answer	Marks	Guidance
c	*Prostanoids:* epoprostenol, iloprost, treprostinil	1	
	Endothelin receptor antagonist: bosentan, ambrisentan, macitentan	1	
	Nitric oxide pathway: nitric oxide, sildenafil, tadalafil	1	Accept 'phosphodiesterase-5 inhibitors'.
	Inodilators: milrinone, enoximone, levosimendan	1	
	Inotropes: dobutamine, dopamine, dopeximine	1	Do NOT accept adrenaline (increases pulmonary hypertension).
d	• Optimise RV preload • Reduce RV afterload • Improve RV contractility • Maintain coronary perfusion pressures	1 1 1 1	
e	• Partial pressure of O_2 • Extracellular pH • Partial pressure of CO_2 • Temperature • Age • Iron status	3	1 mark per correct answer. Can accept PaO_2 and $PaCO_2$.
f	**A** Central venous pulse, 0–8mmHg	1	Can accept values close (within 1–2mmHg) to those listed.
	B Right ventricle, 15–30/0–8mmHg	1	
	C Pulmonary artery, 15–30/4–12mmHg	1	
	D Pulmonary capillary, 2–12mHg	1	

Pulmonary hypertension can cause significant detrimental physiological effects, including acute cardiogenic shock and death. Key concepts in the management are preventing hypoxic pulmonary vasoconstriction to prevent further increases in pulmonary hypertension, as well as offloading the ventricle. Patients typically present with increasing shortness of breath on exertion and should have echocardiography before any operation, be that cardiac or non-cardiac.

Condliffe, R. and Kiely, D. (2017) Critical care management of pulmonary hypertension. *BJA Education*, **17(7):** 228–234.

Elliot, C. and Kiely, D. (2006) Pulmonary hypertension. *CEACCP*, **6(1):** 17–22.

Tarry, D. and Powell, M. (2017) Hypoxic pulmonary vasoconstriction. *BJA Education*, **17(6):** 208–213.

CRQ 5: answer guidance

Syllabus	PA_IS_07, PM_IK_06
Question type	Easy: pass mark 14
Topic	**Chronic post-surgical pain (CPSP)**
Aim	To understand procedures that have a higher incidence of chronic post-surgical pain and the use of pharmacotherapy to control it.
Pass requirements	Correctly elucidate higher centres of pain processing, risk factors for CPSP and strategies to avoid CPSP.

Q	Answer	Marks	Guidance
a	• Amputation (any) • Inguinal hernia repair • Mastectomy • Thoracotomy • Sternotomy • Cholecystectomy	3	1 mark per correct answer.
b	• Psychological vulnerability • Pre-op anxiety • Female • Young age • Genetic predisposition • Previous unpleasant painful experience • Depression • Worker's compensation • Social environment	5	1 mark per correct answer.
c	**Allodynia:** Pain resulting from a stimulus that would not normally cause pain **Hyperalgesia:** Increased pain in response to a stimulus that causes pain	1 1	
d	• Thoracic epidural • Paravertebral block • Erector spinae block • Pectoral nerve block(s) • Serratus anterior plane block • Transverse thoracic plane block	4	1 mark per correct answer. Can accept any reasonable regional technique. PECS1/2 should be considered as 1 block.

Q	Answer	Marks	Guidance
e	*Parecoxib:* COX-2 receptor, antagonist	1	
	Clonidine: alpha-2-adrenergic receptor, agonist	1	
	Ketamine: NMDA-receptor, antagonist	1	
	Gabapentin: voltage-dependent calcium channel, antagonist	1	
f	Spinothalamic tract	1	
g	• Insula • Medial parietal operculum • Mid-cingulate cortex • Periaqueductal grey • Rostroventromedial medulla • Anterior cingulated cortex • Prefrontal cortex • Reticular formation	3	1 mark per correct answer.

Chronic post-surgical pain is probably more common than reported and can be very difficult to manage, often requiring a combination of pharmacological therapy and cognitive behavioural therapy. Pain processing is very complex and is still poorly understood, but anaesthetists should be aware of surgeries and patients that are more likely to develop CPSP. Multimodal pain relief is key here to avoid CPSP in the long term.

Bridges, D., Thompson, S. and Rice, A. (2001) Mechanisms of neuropathic pain. *BJA*, **87(1):** 12–26.

Feizerfan, A. and Sheh, G. (2015) Transition from acute to chronic pain. *CEACCP*, **15(2):** 98–102.

Searle, R. and Simpson, K. (2010) Chronic post-surgical pain. *CEACCP*, **10(1):** 12–14.

Sherwin, A. and Buggy, D. (2018) Anaesthesia for breast surgery. *BJA Education*, **18(11):** 342–348.

CRQ 6: answer guidance

Syllabus	PA_IK_02, PA_IK_14, PA_IS_01, PA_IS_05, PA_IS_06
Question type	Easy: pass mark 12
Topic	**Neonatal resus**
Aim	To recall neonatal anatomy, physiology, pharmacology and the resuscitation of the acutely unwell neonate.
Pass requirements	Correct knowledge of paediatric equipment and neonatal resus algorithm.

Q	Answer	Marks	Guidance
a	• Maternal group B streptococcus • *Listeria monocytogenes* • *Escherichia coli* • *Staphylococcus aureus* • Herpes simplex virus • Enteroviruses • Parechoviruses • *Candida* spp.	3	1 mark per correct answer.
b	Tube size: 3.5mm	1	
	Tube length: 12cm	1	
c	*Atropine:* 80mcg	1	20mcg/kg
	Adrenaline: 40mcg (or 0.4ml of 1:10000 adrenaline)	1	10mcg/kg
	Suxamethonium: 12–16mg	1	3–4mg/kg
	Ketamine: 2–8mg	1	0.5–2mg/kg
	Cefuroxime: 100mg	1	25mg/kg (mg/kg can be accepted)
d	• Initially 10ml/kg crystalloid boluses given	1	Maximum three marks.
	• After 40ml/kg, vasopressors are required	1	
	• Further fluid resuscitation will require 10ml/kg packed red cells	1	
	• Intubation is usually required after 40ml/kg of crystalloids given	1	
e	**CPR ratio:** 15:2.	1	Do not accept 'Antero-lateral' or 'Antero-posterior'.
	Position of defib pads: one pad to the left of the sternum, the other below the left scapula. Alternatively, one pad below right clavicle, the other in the left axilla	1	
	Defib energy: 16J	1	
f	• Large tongue • Large tonsils/adenoids • Subglottic stenosis • Atlanto-axial instability • Micrognathia	4	1 mark per correct answer.

Neonatal resus has a number of key differences to conventional resus, which the anaesthetist should be aware of. Often these patients end up managed in a tertiary neonatal unit but for obvious reasons, can occur anywhere. It is important to keep up to date with the most recent guidelines as they often change.

Ali, U. and Bingham, R. (2018) Current recommendations for paediatric resuscitation. *BJA Education*, **18(4):** 116–121.

Lal, N. and Varshney, T. (2018) The collapsed newborn in the emergency department. *BJA Education*, **18(8):** 254–258.

Melarkode, K. (2009) Anaesthesia for children with Down's syndrome. *Anaesthesia Tutorial of the Week*, **139**.

CRQ 7: answer guidance

Syllabus	SM_IK_01, SM_IK_08
Question type	Medium: pass mark 12
Topic	**Statistics**
Aim	To have an overview knowledge of statistical terms and be able to examine clinical evidence for forms of bias.
Pass requirements	List the phases involved in a clinical trial.

Q	Answer	Marks	Guidance
a	Retrospective studies are used when the disease/item being investigated is rare and using a prospective method would take too long	1	Can also accept when prospective study is unethical.
b	• Difficult to obtain accurate and complete information (recall error) • Not possible to randomise	1 1	Often these studies are inexpensive, as they can utilise existing data, so this is not a possible answer.
c	*Phase 1:* screening for safety; test in small groups of people to identify dose range and side-effects	1	There is also phase 0 which is establishing pharmacodynamics and pharmacokinetics.
	Phase 2: establishing efficacy; usually against placebo or best current treatment; given to larger group of people	1	Can accept different wording as long as basic principle is correct.
	Phase 3: final confirmation of safety and efficacy; given to large group of people to confirm effectiveness	1	
	Phase 4: ongoing evaluation and safety	1	

Q	Answer	Marks	Guidance
d	• Selection bias (e.g. poor randomisation) • Measurement bias (poor measurement outcomes) • Publication bias (journals are more likely to publish positive results; quality of some journals not as good as others) • Commercial bias (bias introduced by funding body) • Attrition bias (subjects who do not complete trial are removed from analysis) • Participation bias (people who are keen to be in studies may show positive results to placebo)	3	1 mark per correct answer. These are the main form of bias. Can accept any other reasonable form of bias or explanation of a type of bias.
e	*Type I error:* a false positive; incorrect rejection of null hypothesis *Type II error:* a false negative; failure to reject a false null hypothesis	1 1	These can be avoided by correct setting of the *P* value and by large sample size. They are inversely related.
f	*Sensitivity:* ability to correctly identify a positive outcome when one exists *Specificity:* ability to identify a negative outcome when one exists *Positive predictive value:* how likely it is that a patient will have the disease/condition being tested for when the result is positive	1 1 1	It is acceptable to use an example in each of the answers to help flesh them out.
g	1a: systematic review of one or more RCT 1b: an RCT 2a: a controlled non-randomised study 2b: a quasi-experimental study (e.g. cohort study) 3: non-experimental study (e.g. case-control) 4: expert opinion.	1 1 1 1	Can accept either 'a/b' answers to gain one mark.
h	A statistical technique that combines the finding of several individual studies on the same topic to reach a single conclusion based on all available evidence	1	

Statistics is often a feared topic for many candidates sitting the final FRCA; however, it is essential as a clinician to be able to understand and interpret many forms of scientific evidence. The curriculum on statistics is actually quite small compared to other areas and so it is worth covering in full. Unfortunately there is no substitute for detailed knowledge of statistics, as it will be clear to an examiner when the candidate is waffling rather than providing a concise answer.

Columb, M. and Atkinson, M. (2016) Statistical analysis: sample size and power estimations. *BJA Education*, **16(5):** 159–161.

Lalkhen, A. and McClusky A. (2008) Statistics V: introduction to clinical trials and systematic reviews. *CEACCP*, **8(4):** 143–146.

McClusky, A. and Lalkhen, A. (2007) Statistics I: data and correlations. *CEACCP*, **7(3):** 95–99.

CRQ 8: answer guidance

Syllabus	PA_IS_06, PR_IK_14
Question type	Easy: pass mark 12
Topic	**Anaphylaxis**
Aim	To be able to competently describe the immediate management of anaphylaxis.
Pass requirements	The immediate management of anaphylaxis and doses.

Q	Answer	Marks	Guidance
a	1 in 11 752	1	Accept between 1 in 10 000 and 1 in 12 000.
b	• Antibiotics (betalactams and glycopeptides) • Neuromuscular blocking agents • Chlorhexidine • Patent blue dye	1 1 1 1	The most common antibiotics were co-amoxiclav and teicoplanin. There were more cases of teicoplanin-related anaphylaxis in NAP6 than co-amoxiclav, but co-amoxiclav was given in more anaesthetics. Other possible causative agents could include sugammadex, latex and iodine; however, these were less common.
c	• Mature B cells produce specific IgE antibodies to allergen (sensitisation phase) • On re-exposure the allergen cross-links two specific IgE receptors, resulting in mast cell degranulation • Release of histamine, tryptase, prostaglandin, leukotriene, TXA2 causes hypotension and clinical manifestation of anaphylaxis	1 1 1	There are three broad parts of the mechanism that must be mentioned for all three marks: sensitisation, degranulation and release of mediators. These all form the clinical picture of anaphylaxis.

Q	Answer	Marks	Guidance
d	• Widespread urticarial rash • Bronchospasm • Cardiovascular collapse/arrest • Swelling of eyelid, lips, tongue • Paradoxical bradycardia	3	1 mark per correct answer. Erythema and urticaria occur due to widespread vasodilation. Cardiac arrhythmias may occur due to widespread activation of the sympathetic nervous system. Less common features may include sweating, goosebumps, nipple erection.
e	• Withdrawal of offending agent • Temporary discontinuation or lightening of anaesthetic agent • Trendelenburg manoeuvre • IV fluid bolus of crystalloid (20ml/kg) • 100% oxygen • Adrenaline (bolus of 100–200mcg IV) • Salbutamol 2.5–5.0mg • IV glucocorticoid (e.g. methylprednisolone 1–2mg/kg, hydrocortisone 200mg)	6	1 mark per correct answer. This should be straightforward management of anaphylaxis. Call for help is not included here, as at final FRCA level one should be expected to be able to instigate immediate management. Calling for skilled assistance may be more appropriate than 'help'. Can accept sugammadex here if it is assumed that rocuronium could be the offending agent. There is no evidence that chlorpheniramine is helpful in acute anaphylaxis, but it may be useful to prevent rebound effect. Noradrenaline/vasopressin can be used in the management of refractory anaphylaxis but not in acute management.
f	0.05mcg/kg/min to 0.1mcg/kg/min	1	This should be started after 2–3 boluses of adrenaline IV.
g	Serum tryptase As soon as possible; at 1–2 hours; at 24 hours	1 1	It is the anaesthetist's responsibility to arrange follow-up with the patient and refer to an allergy clinic/immunologist. It should not be forgotten to send all details to the MHRA via their Yellow Card scheme.

Anaphylaxis in the final FRCA should be considered as low-hanging fruit, and candidates should be able to reel off the management of anaphylaxis easily. NAP6 is surrounding anaphylaxis and is well publicised. There is also good information through the AAGBI, which has a quick reference guide. From a practical point of view, most hospitals will have an 'anaphylaxis box' which will contain all the medications needed as well as a treatment algorithm. Remember that the final FRCA is an exit exam so it is unlikely marks will be given for calling for help; however, this is still a key part of the management.

Cook, T. and Harper, N. (eds) (2018) *NAP6: Anaesthesia, Surgery and Life-Threatening Allergic Reactions*. Royal College of Anaesthetists.

Dewachter, P. and Savic, L. (2019) Perioperative anaphylaxis: pathophysiology, clinical presentation and management. *BJA Education*, **19(10):** 313–320.

CRQ 9: answer guidance

Syllabus	VS_IK_01, VS_IK_05
Question type	Medium: pass mark 12
Topic	**Ruptured abdominal aortic aneurysm**
Aim	To understand the physiological changes at aortic cross-clamping.
Pass requirements	Recall the pitfalls of aggressive fluid resus in the context of a ruptured aneurysm.

Q	Answer	Marks	Guidance
a	• Degradation of elastin fibres • Collagen disruption ultimately causes the rupture • Proteolysis secondary to imbalance in matrix metalloproteinases	2	1 mark per correct answer. Other factors include chronic inflammatory infiltrates, smooth muscle cell apoptosis, increased production of pro-inflammatory cytokines, and can be considered as a mark.
b	Cigarette smoking, male sex, increasing age, COPD, high cholesterol, family history of AAA, cardiovascular disease (IHD/stroke), coexisting connective tissue disease	4	1 mark per correct answer. Age >66 if male and >70 if female.
c	>5.5cm	1	At 5.5cm or above patients should be referred for an opinion by a vascular surgeon within 2 weeks. If it is 3–5.5cm then a less urgent referral is required.
d	• Ruptured viscus • Bowel ischaemia • Acute pancreatitis • Ruptured visceral artery • Ruptured lymphoma • Acute cholecystitis • Strangulated hernia	3	1 mark per correct answer. Most causes of an acute abdomen should be on the differential but if on examination it is pulsatile, this may somewhat narrow. A bedside ultrasound may confirm the diagnosis. Can accept any reasonable answer.

Q	Answer	Marks	Guidance
e	**Glasgow Score:** Age, presence of shock, myocardial disease, cerebrovascular disease, renal disease **Hardman Score:** Age, creatinine (>190µmol/L), haemoglobin (<9g/dl), ischaemia on ECG, a history of loss of consciousness since at hospital	1 + 2	1 mark for score, 1 mark for each variable. These are the two most common scoring systems and are used to predict mortality post surgery.
f	• Dilution of clotting factors • Dilution of haemoglobin and therefore reduction in oxygen-carrying capacity of blood volume • Increase in size of aneurysm • Thrombus disengagement	2	1 mark per correct answer. Over-aggressive fluid resus is associated with poor outcome. In the pre-operative period it may be better to accept a lower MAP.
g	• Increase in afterload • Increased left ventricular end diastolic pressure • Overall reduced cardiac output	2	Grossly there is an increase in afterload and therefore cardiac output decreases. There is a slight change in heart rate to compensate but the longer the cross-clamp is on, the more ischaemic metabolites and inflammatory mediators build, and there is further risk of cardiac depression.
h	20mmHg Anaemia, prolonged hypotension, CPR, hypothermia, severe acidosis, aggressive fluid resuscitation	1 2	The development of compartment syndrome may have negative outcomes such as visceral and renal ischaemia, which could lead to long-term renal damage.

A ruptured abdominal aortic aneurysm is a surgical and anaesthetic emergency. It is important not to fall into the trap of over-aggressive resuscitation in the pre-operative period, as this can have fatal consequences. There are a number of important steps in the management. Firstly at induction patients can lose the tamponade that may be keeping any aneurysm in check. This can again happen at surgical incision. Cross-clamping and removal of cross-clamp can have large physiological implications and the anaesthetist should be prepared to give vasopressors and rapid filling, should the need arise quickly. In reality it is ideal to have two experienced anaesthetists in theatre to manage such cases.

Al-Hashimi, M. and Thompson, J. (2013) Anaesthesia for elective open abdominal aortic aneurysm repair. *CEACCP*, **13(6):** 208–212.

Leonard, A. and Thompson, J. (2008) Anaesthesia for ruptured abdominal aortic aneurysm. *CEACCP*, **8(1):** 11–15.

NICE (2020) *Abdominal aortic aneurysm* [NG156]. Available at: www.nice.org.uk/guidance/ng156 (accessed 2 February 2022).

CRQ 10: answer guidance

Syllabus	EN_IK_01, EN_IS_01, EN_IS_04, DS_IK_02
Question type	Easy: pass mark 12
Topic	**Rhinological surgery**
Aim	To understand the adaptations in anaesthetic technique required for rhinological surgery.
Pass requirements	Describe the basic principles of day surgery and strategies to reduce the risk of bleeding.

Q	Answer	Marks	Guidance
a	• Sleep apnoea (uncontrolled) • Poor functional state • ASA >3 • Uncontrolled/unstable systemic disease (e.g. hypertension, diabetes) • Previous identified high risk of bleeding • Ongoing illness/URTI/LRTI • Team not used to performing this case as a day surgery procedure • Patient refusal • Patient unable to comply with post-operative instructions • Patient has no transport home/no one to stay with them post-operatively • Procedure carries high risk of pain or nausea • Supermorbid obesity	4	1 mark per correct answer. Can accept any reasonable contraindication to day surgery (list is not exhaustive). Obesity or BMI is not usually a contraindication on its own; however, the hospital may be limited by equipment or expertise.
b	• 10–20° head up position • Reverse Trendelenberg position • Low PEEP <5cmH$_2$O	2	1 mark per correct answer. Could accept surgical technique as a possible answer.
c	• Tachycardias • New arrhythmias • Sustained hypertension • Increased risk of myocardial infarction • Increased risk of acute angle-closure glaucoma • Risk of SAH	3	1 mark per correct answer.
d	• Intentional reduction in blood pressure in order to reduce bleeding • MAP to 50–60mmHg • MAP 30% lower than baseline	1 1	Can accept actual value of MAP or degree below baseline.

Q	Answer	Marks	Guidance
e	• Obesity • Predicted difficult airway • Significant acid reflux • Pulmonary disease • OSA • Long duration of surgery • Degree of bleeding (risk of blood aspiration) • Tight control of oxygenation or carbon dioxide clearance	5	1 mark per correct answer.
f	• Use of swab count to include pack • Mark on patient • Part of pack protruding from patient • Pack fixed to airway device • Recording throat pack insertion on swab count board • Throat pack on WHO checklist • Stop before you pack pause • Not using throat pack	4	1 mark per correct answer. It is important to note this is a never event and should be treated as a retained swab.

Questions referencing ENT procedures are commonly encountered in the final examinations because they are often simple procedures which most candidates will be familiar with, but which can be used to examine several themes. A case like this covers day surgery and shared airway in addition to pharmacology and physiology. Questions such as this can also be easily adapted to cover paediatrics.

The use of throat packs is a hot topic. A joint consensus statement (Athanassoglou *et al.*, 2018) resulted in the statement *"The consensus advice, therefore, is that if it is judged that a throat pack is essential, then it should be placed directly by the relevant surgeon (with anaesthetic assistance for laryngoscopy if necessary) as part of the surgical procedure, the pack therefore automatically being part of the surgical swab count"*. However, it is still common practice for anaesthetists to insert throat packs. National Patient Safety Agency guidelines recommend at least one visual check (such as a mark on the patient) and one written check (such as recording insertion and removal on the swab count board).

Athanassoglou, V., Patel, A., Mcguire, B. *et al.* (2018) Systematic review of benefits or harms of routine anaesthetist-inserted throat packs in adults: practice recommendations for inserting and counting throat packs: an evidence-based consensus statement by the Difficult Airway Society (DAS), the British Association of Oral and Maxillofacial Surgeons (BAOMS) and the British Association of Otorhinolaryngology, Head and Neck Surgery (ENT UK). *Anaesthesia*, **73(5):** 612–618.

Bailey, C., Ahuja, M., Bartholomew, K. *et al.* (2019) Guidelines for day-case surgery. *Anaesthesia*, **74(6):** 778–792.

Murdoch, I., Surda, P. and Nguyen-Lu, N. (2021) Anaesthesia for rhinological surgery. *BJA Education*, **21(6):** 225–231.

CRQ 11: answer guidance

Syllabus	AM_IK_08, EN_IK_04
Question type	Easy: pass mark 12
Topic	**OSA**
Aim	To be able to diagnose OSA, understand its underlying pathophysiology and its peri-operative management.
Pass requirements	Understand strategies to change anaesthetic practice for an OSA patient.

Q	Answer	Marks	Guidance
a	• Obesity • Age (40–70 years) • Male • Excess alcohol intake • Smoking • Pregnancy • Sedentary lifestyle • Unemployment • Neck circumference >40cm • Craniofacial abnormalities • Neuromuscular disease • Tonsillar/adenoid hypertrophy	6	1 mark per correct answer.
b	• Negative pressure during inspiration causes oropharyngeal collapse • Decreased oropharyngeal muscle tone • Increased fatty deposits cause narrowing of oropharynx	2	1 mark per correct answer. 'Airway collapse' should not be accepted on its own, as it is more of a consequence than part of the pathophysiology.
c	• STOP BANG questionnaire • Sleep polysomnography • Oxygen desaturation index • High clinical suspicion	2	1 mark per correct answer. Should not accept 'sleep studies' as this is not necessarily true, must include the word 'polysomnography'.
d	Mild: AHI >5	1	
	Moderate: AHI >15	1	
	Severe: AHI >30	1	
e	• Decreased frequency of cardiac arrhythmias • Improved cardiac function • Reduced platelet aggregation • Reduced cardiovascular events • Reduced cerebrovascular events • Improved daytime sleepiness • Improved quality of life • Reduced depression	4	1 mark per correct answer. Can accept reduced risk of either MI or stroke.

Q	Answer	Marks	Guidance
f	• Use short-acting sedative agents • Use of regional/local anaesthetic techniques • Fully reverse neuromuscular blockade • Supplementary oxygen post-operatively • Recommence CPAP post-operatively	3	1 mark per correct answer. Could also accept the avoidance of sedative agents. If individual drugs are given, then this should only be 1 mark total.

OSA is becoming increasingly common in the general population and it can have significant and life-changing effects in the long term. Importantly, in the peri-operative phase, good anaesthetic and post-operative management can reduce complications. The mainstay of treatment of OSA is lifestyle modification, but also CPAP can be used. Often this should be carried with the patient throughout their surgical journey and should be placed on the patient post-operatively. Perhaps a contraindication to this would be upper airway surgery and an MDT-style approach with the operating surgeon should be taken to manage these patients.

Hall, A. (2015) Sleep physiology and the perioperative care of patients with sleep disorders. *BJA Education*, **15(4):** 167–172.

Martinez, G. and Faber, P. (2011) Obstructive sleep apnoea. *CEACCP*, **11(1):** 5–8.

CRQ 12: answer guidance

Syllabus	PR_IK_16, CT_IK_01
Question type	Hard: pass mark 10
Topic	**Anaesthesia for lung transplantation**
Aim	To understand the indications and contraindications for lung transplant as well as the peri-operative management.
Pass requirements	List the clinical features of primary graft dysfunction.

Q	Answer	Marks	Guidance
a	• Idiopathic interstitial pneumonia • COPD • Cystic fibrosis	2	1 mark per correct answer. These are the most common causes.
b	• Chronic end-stage lung disease that has a >50% risk of death within 2 years • But have a high probability of surviving >5 years with transplant	1 1	These are the physiological characteristics; however, there may be variations on this that could be patient-specific.

Q	Answer	Marks	Guidance
c	• Recent malignancy • Acute unstable medical condition • Uncontrolled bleeding • Significant dysfunction in another major organ • Chronic uncontrolled multi-drug-resistant infection (e.g. TB) • BMI >35 • Significant chest wall or spinal deformity • Alcohol or drug abuse • Psychological condition meaning patient is uncooperative • Non-adherence to medical therapy • Limited rehab potential • Lack of a support team	4	1 mark per correct answer. Relative contraindications include: age >65 (with poor reserve), BMI >30, malnutrition, mechanical ventilation, hepatitis, HIV, atherosclerotic disease, poorly controlled diabetes, previous chest surgery.
d	• V/Q scan: to identify the least functional lung • TTE: to evaluate right heart function and pulmonary artery pressure • CT chest: to rule out occult malignancy/potency of great vessels/lung collaterals • Right heart catheter: to evaluate pulmonary artery pressure • Pulmonary function tests: to evaluate pre-operative lung function and suitability for transplant	4	Patients who present for lung transplant often have other comorbidities. Most investigations are focused around residual lung function (to determine one-lung vs. two-lung transplant) or right heart function. Must include test and rationale for 1 mark.
e	• Severe pulmonary hypertension • Patient already on ECMO	1 1	In centres that perform most cases off-pump these are the main indications for changing to on-pump.
f	5.5 hours or greater	1	Ischaemia time of >5.5 hours is associated with increased risk. Therefore anaesthesia is carefully timed (1 hour for induction, 1 hour surgical time planned before ischaemia). Accept between 4 and 6 hours.
g	Severe pulmonary hypertension	1	Anaesthetists should be wary of all patients with severe pulmonary hypertension, as this can lead not only to graft failure but also other on-table complications.
h	• Impaired oxygenation • Diffuse opacities on chest radiograph	1 1	These two features define primary graft dysfunction so should be identified early.

CRQs and SBAs for the Final FRCA

Q	Answer	Marks	Guidance
i	• Calcineurin inibitors (ciclosporin/tacrolimus) • Antiproliferative agent (azathioprine/mycophenolate) • Corticosteroids	2	1 mark per correct answer. A combination of these drugs is used for anti-rejection. All of these can have system-wide complications, so outside of the transplant surgery they should be screened for. It would be enough in this question to have the class only.

Lung transplant surgery is something that most candidates would not have seen during their anaesthetic career, but the basic principles are similar to those of thoracic surgery in patients with underlying respiratory disease. Most of these patients will present with end-stage lung disease so anaesthetists must be wary of other coexisting diseases such as vascular and coronary disease. The key part in the management of lung transplant patients is selection of the correct patients. There are also a variety of contraindications that one should be familiar with. These patients may also present for surgery later on in their lives, so it is important to have an understanding of the immunosuppressive regime as well as some of the complications that may be encountered with them.

Buckwell, E., Vickery, B. and Sidebotham, D. (2020) Anaesthesia for lung transplantation. *BJA Education*, **20(11):** 368–376.

SBA 1: answer = B – Motor function

Local anaesthetic blockade is dependent on concentration. The most susceptible fibres are the A-gamma spindle efferents and the A-delta nociceptive fibres. The least susceptible are the C-fibres, which are unmyelinated. The discrepancy in LA blockade is evident following an epidural top-up – whereby sympathetic tone is the first to be lost, followed by pain/cold sensation, and then proprioception. Motor function (assessed by the Bromage score) is the last to be lost. The sensation of touch and proprioception, carried by A-beta fibres, is the second-to-last modality to be lost and may be distressing to patients if not well explained.

Taylor, A. and McLeod, G. (2020) Basic pharmacology of local anaesthetics. *BJA Education*, **20(2):** 34–41.

SBA 2: answer = D – Mueller's syndrome

Mueller's syndrome is one of the signs of a successful stellate ganglion block, characterised by an ipsilateral warmth of the face and injection of the ipsilateral tympanic membrane. The other options are all possible complications due to needling or injection.

Menon, R. and Swanepoel, A. (2015) Sympathetic blocks. *CEACCP*, **10(3):** 88–92.

SBA 3: answer = B – AFOI and bronchial blocker

This patient has a predicted difficult airway and is presenting for a non-emergency procedure. The safest way to proceed with this procedure is to secure the airway with an awake fibre-optic intubation. Using a standard Robertshaw double-lumen tube is likely to be unsuccessful, as the rigidity and shape of the tube will not navigate the nasal passage. Therefore performing an AFOI with bronchial blockers is the safest and easiest way to facilitate the surgery.

Ng, A. and Swanevelder, J. (2010) Hypoxaemia during one-lung anaesthesia. *CEACCP*, **(10)4:** 117–122.

SBA 4: answer = A – Digital subtraction angiography (DSA) of the brain

The patient has a probable cerebral aneurysm which at this stage is likely to be unruptured. Although a CT head is likely to be the first choice of imaging due to its availability, the gold standard investigation of choice would be a digital subtraction angiography. MRA would also be useful but due to the longer scanning time and limited availability it is currently not considered as the gold standard.

Patel, S. and Reddy, U. (2016) Anaesthesia for interventional neuroradiology. *BJA Education*, **16(5):** 147–152.

SBA 5: answer = B – Thread the catheter and use it as an intrathecal catheter

Although intrathecal catheters can be variable in their efficacy and are associated with a higher number of complications, it is the most appropriate option here. The patient has had many attempts at an epidural and removing the needle and performing another epidural increases the risk of further complications, including additional dural puncture. IV pain relief is unlikely to be as effective. A low dose CSE would not be possible in this situation.

Sharpe, P. (2001) Accidental dural puncture in obstetrics. *CEACCP*, **1(3):** 81–84.

SBA 6: answer = C – The trachealis muscle forms the posterior wall of the trachea

The trachealis muscle forms the posterior wall, while 16–20 C-shaped cartilaginous rings form the anterior wall. The trachea ends at level T4/T5 in a supine patient but this may change in an upright patient due to the effect of gravity. The lingular segments are part of the left lung due to the presence of the heart. There are 10 bronchopulmonary segments of the right lung.

Kabadayi, S. and Bellamy, M. (2017) Bronchoscopy in critical care. *BJA Education*, **17(2):** 48–56.

SBA 7: answer = C – CO_2 (far infrared 10600nm)

The CO_2 (gas) lasing medium is used as a laser scalpel for cutting and coagulation of soft tissue that primarily contains water – including laryngeal tissue. Argon is more commonly used in dermatological or ophthalmic settings, Ho:YAG is commonly used in lithotripsy or sinus surgery, and Nd:YAG in GI bleeding. Ruby is less commonly used clinically, but is seen in hair removal/tattoo removal.

Pearson, K. and McGuire, B. (2017) Anaesthesia for laryngo-tracheal surgery, including tubeless field techniques. *BJA Education*, **17(7):** 242–248.

Simpson, E. (2012) The basic principles of laser technology, uses and safety measures in anaesthesia. *Anaesthesia Tutorial of the Week*, **255**.

SBA 8: answer = E – 12960ml

The Parkland formula is used to calculate fluid *replacement* following burns. For the first 24 hours the needs are: 4ml × total body surface area (%) × body weight (kg). 50% of this fluid should be given in the first 8 hours, and the rest in the following 16 hours. Actual fluid *resuscitation* is guided by urine output. To calculate the body surface area the 'rule of nines' is used. In this case it is 9% for each limb, 18% for chest and stomach and 4.5% for the face. This works out to 12960ml over 24 hours.

Bishop, S. and Maguire, S. (2012) Anaesthesia and intensive care for major burns. *CEACCP*, **12(3):** 118–122.

SBA 9: answer = D – Carbamazepine

This patient demonstrates the classic symptoms of trigeminal neuralgia, as well as having multiple sclerosis which is an independent risk factor. The first-line pharmacotherapy agent is carbamazepine (NNT 1.8). Other anticonvulsants could be used but are not considered as the first-line. Surgical decompression has good efficacy but due to complications and the complexity of the surgery, pharmacological treatment should be trialled first.

Vasappa, C., Kappur, S. and Krovvidi, H. (2016) Trigeminal neuralgia. *BJA Education*, **16(10):** 353–356.

SBA 10: answer = C – Start prostaglandin infusion

Cyanosis in this case occurs when the ductus arteriosus is closed, which can temporarily be reversed by an infusion of prostaglandin E2. A balloon atrial septostomy can also be performed to allow a greater mixing at the level of the atria; however, this would need more time and expertise. Surgical correction can be performed at a later date under elective conditions after initial stabilisation. Nitrate infusions have no benefit in this case, nor does immediate ventilation and intubation.

Murphy, P. (2005) The fetal circulation. *CEACCP*, **5(4):** 107–112.

SBA 11: answer = A – Interventional radiology-guided chest drain

The patient has an exudative pleural tap due to low pH, glucose of 1mmol/L and pH of 7.1 according to Light's criteria, therefore IV diuretics are unlikely to have an effect. If the tap contained food particles, this may be suggestive of oesophageal rupture and this would require a thoracics referral. The results are highly suggestive of an empyema, the best management of which would be an IR-guided chest drain. This provides accurate source control, which will be used in combination with intravenous antibiotics. A Seldinger chest drain is unlikely to successfully target the empyema. If this was malignant then the patient should have a staging CT and this would likely have an amylase level of >110U/L.

Walters, J., Foley, N. and Molyneux, M. (2011) Pus in the thorax: management of empyema and lung abscesses. *CEACCP*, **11(6):** 229–233.

SBA 12: answer = A – Stop the surgery

The patient must be assumed to be having a peri-operative myocardial infarction until this can be excluded. The immediate management will be to stop the surgery and aim to stop any precipitating factors. The patient should receive 100% oxygen acutely, although it is not appropriate to over-oxygenate the patient. IV GTN may be the next step in the management while a full 12-lead ECG is being performed. Deepening the plane of anaesthesia may be appropriate as long as the patient does not show any signs of being haemodynamically unstable, as a light plane of anaesthesia could precipitate an intra-operative MI.

Priebe, H. (2005) Perioperative myocardial infarction – aetiology and prevention. *BJA*, **95(1):** 3–19.

SBA 13: answer = E – Cold compress

In the event of extravasation there are a number of drugs that have the potential to cause tissue damage or injury, one of which is sodium bicarbonate. The aim of treatment should be to dilute and spread the pharmacological agent. This will prevent vasoconstriction and direct toxicity. A cold compress should be avoided as this may cause further vasoconstriction and tissue damage. Saline washout will dilute any pharmacological agent. Although liposuction (aspiration of fat and extravasated material) can also be used, this is less effective and far less practical. Hyaluronidase makes tissue more permeable, and steroids may have an anti-inflammatory effect.

Lake, C. and Beecroft, C. (2010) Extravasation injuries and accidental intra-arterial injection. *CEACCP*, **10(4):** 109–113.

SBA 14: answer = C – Cardiac disease

Between 2016 and 2018 there were 217 maternal deaths in the UK (9.7 deaths per 100 000). The most common cause of death was cardiac disease (23% or 50 women), with the next most common being VTE. Patients who present antenatally with signs of heart disease such as chest pain or shortness of breath on exertion should be referred for echocardiography to elucidate the nature of their cardiac disease, and they will need an individualised labour and delivery plan as they approach the end of their pregnancy.

MBRRACE-UK (2020) *Saving Lives, Improving Mothers' Care*: Executive Summary. Available at: www.npeu.ox.ac.uk/assets/downloads/mbrrace-uk/reports/maternal-report-2020/MBRRACE-UK_Maternal_Report_Dec_2020_-_Ex_Summary_v10.pdf (accessed 5 February 2022).

SBA 15: answer = D – Morphine

Propofol and opioids have the least effect on MEPs and SSEPs. Therefore, TIVA with propofol and remifentanil tends to be the anaesthetic of choice for this procedure. However, an increased dose of propofol can reduce the amplitude of EPs. Sevoflurane (as well as other halogenated volatile agents) decreases EP amplitude and increases latency, whereas nitrous oxide and midazolam only reduce EP amplitude. Ketamine causes an increase in EP amplitude.

Lucile Packard Children's Hospital, Stanford (2016) *Guidelines for the anaesthetic management of patients with scoliosis undergoing posterior spinal fusion surgery.* Available at http://med.stanford.edu/content/dam/sm/pedsanesthesia/documents/GuidelinesfortheAnesthetic Managemenof PatientsUndergoingSpinalFusionSurgery%2011-4-16.pdf (accessed 5 February 2022).

Nowicki, R. (2014) Anaesthesia for major spinal surgery. *CEACCP*, **14(4):** 147–152.

SBA 16: answer = B – Paravertebral block

Both thoracic epidural and paravertebral block have been found to be equal with regard to post-operative pain relief, but the paravertebral block has been associated with fewer side-effects (e.g. hypotension and post-operative chest infection (PROSPECT trial)). Intrathecal opiates are unlikely to offer long duration pain relief and a PCA is not likely to achieve gold standard pain relief. Intercostal blocks can be useful and will provide good pain relief, but in a localised area only.

Mesbah, A., Yeung, J. and Gao, F. (2015) Pain after thoracotomy. *BJA Education*, **16(1):** 1–7.

SBA 17: answer = B – Prilocaine 40mg

Prilocaine, heavy bupivacaine (Marcaine), levobupivacaine (Chirocaine), and 2-chloroprocaine are the only local anaesthetic agents approved for intrathecal use in the UK. Note that plain bupivacaine is not licensed for intrathecal use, despite its continued use. Low dose (<10mg) Marcaine and Chirocaine has been attempted for ambulatory surgery, but still demonstrates prolonged recovery times. Prilocaine 40–60mg is more appropriate for lower limb/lower abdominal procedures lasting no more than 90 minutes (note that doses above 50mg are not licensed in the UK for intrathecal administration).

Rattenbery, W., Hertling, A. and Erskine, R. (2019) Spinal anaesthesia for ambulatory surgery. *BJA Education*, **19(10):** 321–328.

SBA 18: answer = C – Right coronary artery

The patient is having an inferior myocardial infarction, which accounts for around 40–50% of all myocardial infarctions. The most likely artery involved is the right coronary artery (RCA), which is dominant in around 80% of patients. An inferior MI carries a more favourable mortality providing it is diagnosed and treated swiftly.

Reed-Poysden, C. and Gupta, K. (2015) Acute coronary syndromes. *BJA Education*, **15(6):** 286–293.

SBA 19: answer = E – Tracheobronchial stenting

All of these are methods of managing cancerous airway lesions. To avoid damage to, or displacement of tracheobronchial stents, great care must be taken when instrumenting the airway and therefore fibre-optic intubation must always be used.

Nethercott, D., Strang, T. and Krysiak, P. (2012) Airway stents: anaesthetic implications. *BJA Education*, **10(2):** 53–58.

SBA 20: answer = A – The patient should continue warfarin with no change to target INR

Current joint guidance from the Royal College of Anaesthetists and Royal College of Ophthalmologists suggests that anticoagulants and antiplatelets should be continued in the peri-operative period for cataract surgery. This is because the risk of thrombotic events is greater than the risk of bleeding in high-risk patients. Although it would be safe to bridge these patients with heparin, it is not necessary. There is no reason for pre-operative tranexamic acid, and stopping warfarin would be an unnecessary risk. 92-year-old patients are likely to be at high risk for general anaesthesia, so this should be avoided.

Anker, R. and Kaur, N. (2016) Regional anaesthesia for ophthalmic surgery. *BJA Education*, **17(7):** 221–227.

SBA 21: answer = B – Muscle atrophy in affected limb

The Budapest criteria are used in the diagnosis of complex regional pain syndrome. Patients need to have continuous pain with no other aetiology, that is disproportionate in its intensity. They must also have one symptom in each of the four categories (sensory, vasomotor, sudomotor/oedema, and motor/trophic), and at least one sign in two or more of the aforementioned categories. Although there may be motor dysfunction of the affected limb, CRPS is not associated directly with muscle atrophy and therefore it is not a part of the Budapest criteria.

Bharwani, K., Dirckx, M. and Huygen, F. (2017) Complex regional pain syndrome: diagnosis and treatment. *BJA Education*, **17(8):** 262–268.

SBA 22: answer = A – Apert syndrome

Apert syndrome is associated with midface hypoplasia and although bag-mask ventilation may be difficult, intubation is not affected. Conversely, Treacher Collins syndrome and Pierre Robin sequence are associated with difficult intubation, with bag-mask ventilation usually possible. Orofacial clefts do not cause difficult airways alone, but are often associated with other pathology. Gaucher disease is an inborn error of metabolism and is not usually associated with airway manifestations.

Prasad, Y. (2012) The difficult paediatric airway. *Anaesthesia Tutorial of the Week*, **250**.

Raj, D. and Luginbuehl, I. (2015) Managing the difficult airway in the syndromic child. *CEACCP*, **15(1):** 7–13.

Somerville, N. and Fenlon, S. (2005) Anaesthesia for cleft lip and palate surgery. *CEACCP*, **5(3):** 76–79.

SBA 23: answer = C – 1g/kg fat

The body requires 1g/kg fat per 24h as a basal metabolic requirement, but in critical illness this may increase. The body requires 30ml/kg water, 1–2mmol/kg of sodium and potassium, 0.1mmol/kg calcium and magnesium and 0.2–0.5mmol/kg phosphate. In terms of energy, the patient will also require 2g/kg carbohydrate and 0.8–1.2g/kg protein.

Chowdhury, R. and Lobaz, S. (2019) Nutrition in critical care. *BJA Education*, **19(3):** 90–95.

SBA 24: answer = E – IV calcium gluconate

ECG features of hypocalcaemia are common after a massive transfusion. This is because the citrate contained within the stored blood products chelates calcium, resulting in hypotension. Hyperkalaemia is less common in massive transfusions, unless the patient is also acidotic and hypothermic. Hypothermia should also be avoided during transfusion due to the risk of developing further coagulopathy. Acidosis from blood transfusion is due to high storage levels of lactic acid, but is normally rectified by adequate fluid replacement. There is no role for sodium bicarbonate in this situation.

Maxwell, M. and Wilson, M. (2006) Complications of blood transfusion. *BJA Education*, **6(6):** 225–229.

SBA 25: answer = A – Mu

As well as having the greatest effect on supra-spinal and spinal analgesia, the mu receptor is also most implicated in respiratory depression. It is also responsible for the feeling of euphoria associated with opioid administration. There is no gamma opioid receptor.

McDonald, J. and Lambert, D. (2015) Opioid receptors. *BJA Education*, **15(5):** 219–224.

SBA 26: answer = D – Noradrenaline

Noradrenaline is recommended as the first-line vasopressor. Ephedrine increases uteroplacental blood flow, but results in foetal acidosis. AVP is uterotonic, and thus avoided. Dobutamine has beneficial properties when used in conjunction with noradrenaline. Adrenaline is reserved for resuscitation and it is tocolytic.

Banerjee, A. and Cantellow, S. (2021) Maternal critical care: part I. *BJA Education*, **21(4):** 140–147.

SBA 27: answer = D – Vomiting twice since injury

Vomiting more than once after a head injury is listed by NICE as an indication for head CT in adult patients. Presence or absence of a head wound is not an indication for adults. Age is a consideration but the cut-off is 65 or older. This lady has a GCS of 14 on initial assessment in the ED; the cut-off is less than 13. However, if after 2 hours in the ED the GCS is not back to 15, this is an indication for head CT. Dangerous mechanism of injury is only an indication for CT in conjunction with loss of consciousness or amnesia (at any point since the injury).

NICE (2014, updated 2019) *Head injury: assessment and early management* [CG176].

SBA 28: answer = D – 10.1%

This patient has a Lee's revised risk score of 2 (1 point for previous TIA and 1 point for pathological Q waves on ECG). He does not score for hypertension or oral tablet-controlled anti-diabetic agents. This correlates to a 10.1% risk for MI, cardiac arrest or death 30 days following non-cardiac surgery. This score was updated in 2017 to include 5 high quality external variations, which gave a higher risk than the original 1999 score (see reference) and is now widely accepted.

Duceppe, E., Parlow, J., MacDonald, P. *et al.* (2017) Canadian Cardiovascular Society guidelines on preoperative cardiac risk assessment and management for patients who undergo non-cardiac surgery. *Canadian Journal of Cardiology*, **33(1):** 17–32.

Minto, G. and Biccard, B. (2014) Assessment of the high-risk peri-operative patient. *CEACCP*, **14(1):** 12–17.

SBA 29: answer = D – Use of mild sedation

The national consensus, supported by *WHO surgical safety checklist supporting information* (2009) is that the only mark on the patient should be placed by the surgical team. Any additional mark placed in relation to the block risks introducing error. Although the debate continues surrounding use of sedation for blocks, mild sedation – which maintains verbal contact with the patient – is less likely to introduce error in this situation.

Topor, B., Oldman, M. and Nicholls, B. (2020) Best practices for safety and quality in peripheral regional anaesthesia. *BJA Education*, **20(10):** 341–347.

SBA 30: answer = A – Corrected flow time (FTc)

The corrected flow time most accurately represents the preload of the left ventricle. The normal value is 0.33–0.36 seconds. This corresponds to the duration of time that there is flow from the left ventricle during systole. A low FTc normally correlates to a reduced preload, and these patients should receive a fluid challenge. Peak velocity and mean acceleration are related to the contractility of the ventricle. Cycle time is a variable related to the heart rate. Minute distance is the distance blood moves down the aorta in one minute.

Drummond, K. and Murphy, E. (2012) Minimally invasive cardiac output monitors. *CEACCP*, **12(1):** 5–10.

SBA 31: answer = E – Lidocaine 9mg/kg without adrenaline

Lidocaine is the most commonly used local anaesthetic agent for topicalisation of the airway. Contrary to perineural doses, the maximum safe dose for topicalisation is 9mg/kg, although this is rarely required. This accounts for the proportion of local anaesthetic that will be ingested.

Leslie, D. and Stacey, M. (2014) Awake intubation. *CEACCP*, **15(2):** 64–67.

Pearson, K. and McGuire, B. (2017) Anaesthesia for laryngo-tracheal surgery, including tubeless field techniques. *BJA Education*, **17(7):** 242–248.

SBA 32: answer = B – Retro-bulbar haemorrhage

A retro-bulbar haemorrhage typically presents with proptosis and signs of raised intraocular pressure. This complication can occur rarely after a peribulbar block, with abnormal coagulation and a 'moving field' being risk factors. Patients with AF are likely to be on anticoagulant medication. The haemorrhage may need an emergency lateral canthotomy or decompression if it progresses. Ecchymosis is periorbital bruising and normally self-limiting. Globe injury would result in sudden pain and visual acuity changes but no proptosis, as would optic nerve atrophy. Muscular palsy would more likely give rise to ptosis and diplopia.

Anker, R. and Kaur, N. (2017) Regional anaesthesia for ophthalmic surgery. *BJA Education*, **17(7):** 221–227.

SBA 33: answer = C – 90mg of modified release oral morphine – BD regularly, and 20mg of immediate release oral morphine 4-hourly PRN

Safe and appropriate conversion of IV opioids to oral opioids is necessary to avoid under- and over-dosing. The equation used for this conversion is:
(1) Oral equivalent dose = IV dose over 24 hours multiplied by 2 or 3 (as dictated by equipotency of oral vs. IV morphine).
(2) 50% of oral total dose taken, and given as a BD preparation.
(3) 1/6th of the oral total dose taken, and used as the PRN dose for immediate release morphine 4-hourly.

In this case, the maximum oral dose will be 120–180mg. 50% is therefore 60–90mg. The PRN dose will be 20–30mg 4-hourly.

Simpson, G. and Jackson, M. (2017) Perioperative management of opioid-tolerant patients. *BJA Education*, **17(4):** 124–128.

SBA 34: answer = C – 6 hours

Bowel prep is considered a thickened fluid and so will be considered food. Therefore, a minimum starvation time of 6 hours for elective surgery is recommended prior to anaesthesia, to reduce the risk of pulmonary aspiration.

Frykholm, P., Schindler, E., Sümpelmann, R., Walker, R. and Weiss, M. (2017) Preoperative fasting in children: review of existing guidelines and recent developments. *BJA*, **120(3):** 469–474.

SBA 35: answer = D – Shortened QTc

The patient is severely hypercalcaemic, most likely from the underlying malignancy with metastases. The most likely ECG change in severe hypercalcaemia is a shortened QT interval, which may progress into the formation of J waves (Osborn waves). The main treatment in this case would commence with aggressive fluid rehydration. Bisphosphonates could be considered in hypercalcaemia with an underlying malignancy, if fluid therapy is not successful.

Parikh, M. and Webb, S. (2012) Cations: potassium, calcium and magnesium. *CEACCP*, **12(4):** 195–198.

SBA 36: answer = A – Permanent pacemaker insertion

The patient has second-degree AV block (Mobitz Type II block), which has a high risk of manifesting into third-degree heart block and subsequent cardiac arrest – especially peri-operatively. Even though the patient is asymptomatic, they should have a permanent pacemaker inserted. If the surgery was emergency surgery they may have a temporary pacing wire inserted, followed by a permanent pacemaker later on. The patient requires some form of intervention rather than further testing at this stage.

Dua, N. and Kumra, V. (2007) Management of peri-operative arrhythmias. *Indian Journal of Anaesthesia*, **51(4):** 310–323.

SBA 37: answer = D – Tolcapone

Tolcapone is a COMT inhibitor and prevents the breakdown of dopamine, therefore increasing its availability at the synaptic cleft. Other drugs are also metabolised by the same pathway (e.g. adrenaline) and so dose adjustments may need to be made. It is also important to reinstate anti-parkinsonian medication as soon as possible after surgery. If the patient is unable to swallow after surgery, they may need conversion of their regular medication to a rotigotine patch or to IV apomorphine (both dopamine agonists). Selegiline is a monoamine oxidase B inhibitor.

Chambers, D., Sebastian, J. and Ahearn, D. (2017) Parkinson's disease. *BJA Education*, **17(4):** 145–149.

SBA 38: answer = D – Stop oxytocin infusion

The aim of intrauterine foetal resuscitation is to improve oxygen delivery and alleviate foetal distress. While preparations for emergency delivery are made, intrauterine foetal resuscitation can buy time to allow a regional anaesthetic approach to be considered. The steps necessary are:
(1) Relieve aortocaval compression
(2) Stop uterotonics (oxytocin in this case)
(3) Tocolysis
(4) 100% O_2 via a non-rebreathe mask
(5) Maternal cardiovascular support.

As the concern is related to uterine hyperstimulation, stopping oxytocin is an important first step.

Iradakuna, C., Lambert, B. and Moreiras, J. (2010) Resuscitation of the newborn. *Anaesthesia Tutorial of the Week*, **167**.

SBA 39: answer = E – Induction with propofol and remifentanil and insertion of supraglottic airway

The most appropriate strategy would be an IV induction with propofol, remifentanil and insertion of a supraglottic airway. This will allow the patient to be woken up during the surgery after a scalp block has been performed and Mayfield pins are in place with minimal coughing and gagging. The use of an ET tube may cause the patient to cough in the waking phase and should be avoided in these cases. Sedation and block is not appropriate, as the placement of the Mayfield pins is significantly stimulating and should not be performed under block alone.

Burnard, C. and Sebastian, J. (2014) Anaesthesia for awake craniotomy. *BJA Education*, **14(1):** 6–11.

SBA 40: answer = E – Severe left ventricular dysfunction with severe cardio-hepatic liver dysfunction

Severe liver or renal dysfunction are contraindications to transplantation. The other answers could all be indications for transplant.

Edwards, S., Allen, S. and Sidebotham, D. (2021) Anaesthesia for heart transplantation. *BJA Education*, **21(8):** 284–291.

SBA 41: answer = E – Epidural with catheter

Within the AoA guidelines, various blocks are stratified according to risk. Central neuraxial blockade carries the highest risk of significant complications, with catheter techniques thought to confer lowest risk.

Harrop-Griffiths, W. (2013) Guidelines: patients with abnormalities of coagulation. *Anaesthesia*, **68:** 966–972.

SBA 42: answer = E – Radiation

Radiation corresponds to the highest proportion of heat loss intra-operatively (40%). Convection contributes to 30%, evaporation 15%, respiration 10% and conduction 5%. General and regional anaesthesia causes a 0.5–1.0°C drop in core temperature in the first hour of an operation, and 0.3°C for each hour thereafter.

Sullivan, G. and Edmondson, C. (2008) Heat and temperature. *CEACCP*, **8(3):** 104–107.

SBA 43: answer = B – Neural integrity monitor

This monitors recurrent laryngeal nerve integrity: unilateral damage results in a hoarse voice due to unopposed action of cricothyroid muscle. Bilateral injury results in inability to abduct the cords, and severe stridor. This necessitates a tracheostomy.

Ahmed-Nusrath, A. (2017) Anaesthesia for head and neck cancer surgery. *BJA Education*, **17(12):** 383–389.

SBA 44: answer = B – Continue with the surgery on aspirin and clopidogrel

Having surgery soon after an MI that required stent insertion should be avoided, but in this case the patient has critical stenosis (>70%) with symptoms of TIA. Therefore, pausing the surgery is not an option. The patient will need to continue both antiplatelet agents to prevent the risk of myocardial thrombosis and accept the bleeding risk. Continuing only aspirin is likely to be ineffective so soon after stent placement. Switching the patient to any heparin preparation is also likely to be ineffective in preventing thrombosis around the stent.

Oprea, A. and Popescu, W. (2013) Perioperative management of anti-platelet therapy. *BJA*, **11(1):** i3–i17.

SBA 45: answer = E – Keogh's manoeuvre

A reaction to >3 provocative tests mean that sacroiliac joint dysfunction is the likely source of pain. Tests include compression test, distraction test, Patrick's sign, Gaenslen test, thigh thrust test, Fortin's finger test and Gillet test. If >3 tests are positive, a diagnostic SIJ injection is performed, with a good response being a reduction in pain of >70% which could last up to 1 year.

Sandrasegram, N., Gupta, R. and Baloch, M. (2020) Diagnosis and management of sacrococcygeal pain. *BJA Education*, **20(3):** 74–79.

SBA 46: answer = B – 18ml

Circumcision requires a block to T10. As per the Armitage formula for dosing in caudal anaesthesia, this would require 1ml/kg of 0.25% bupivacaine. Using 0.5ml/kg will get a sacral block only and using 1.25ml/kg will get a higher than needed block and may lead to complications. When dosing, it is important to not exceed the toxic levels for bupivacaine (2.5mg/kg).

Gandhi, M. and Vashisht, R. (2010) Anaesthesia for paediatric urology. *CEACCP*, **10(5):** 152–157.

SBA 47: answer = D – Abandon the procedure

There are a variety of reasons that the patient may become hypoxic. As the procedure is semi-elective to aid respiratory weaning (rather than for an emergency reason), it is most sensible to abandon the procedure and re-evaluate at a later time once the patient has stabilised.

Batuwitage, B., Webber, S. and Glossop, A. (2014) Percutaneous tracheostomy. *CEACCP*, **14(6):** 268–272.

SBA 48: answer = E – Abdominal compartment syndrome

Abdominal compartment syndrome is more likely following major abdominal surgery where primary closure has been achieved, but tightly. It is also associated with massive transfusion and a high BMI along with a number of other risk factors (see reference). A high intra-abdominal pressure causes reduced perfusion to the renal system via direct compression of the renal vasculature, and hypercarbia due to reduced ventilation secondary to diaphragmatic splinting. Bowel injury is possible in this scenario, but less likely. The patient may also be hypovolaemic, but this would not commonly give rise to abdominal pain. Surgical dehiscence occurs later, and would not necessarily cause hypercarbia. It would be too early to see such severe signs of ventilator-associated pneumonia.

Berry, N. and Fletcher, S. (2012) Abdominal compartment syndrome. *CEACCP*, **12(3):** 110–117.

SBA 49: answer = C – Ethanol

This is a high anion gap acidosis. The anion gap is calculated via: $(Na^+ + K^+) - (Cl^- + HCO_3^-)$. In this patient it is therefore $(140 + 4.5) - (108 + 10) = 27.5$. The normal value for the anion gap is 8–16mmol/L. The history of fluctuating consciousness and location she was found suggest that this could be a case of ethylene glycol poisoning (antifreeze). The acidosis is caused by metabolism of ethylene glycol by alcohol dehydrogenase, which can cause neurological damage and eventually death. Ethanol has a greater affinity for alcohol dehydrogenase so can be used in the acute treatment of ethylene glycol poisoning. If this is unsuccessful or unavailable, then CVVHF could be an option. The patient does not have DKA or hyperkalaemia so does not need insulin. Sodium bicarbonate is likely to treat only the acidosis but not necessarily the underlying cause.

Ward, C. and Sair, M. (2010) Oral poisoning: an update. *CEACCP*, **10(1):** 6–11.

SBA 50: answer = A – Open surgery is preferred to laparoscopy

Non-obstetric surgery in pregnant patients requires careful thought for both maternal and foetal considerations. Minimally invasive and laparoscopic approaches are preferred for abdominal surgery. Aortocaval compression is noted from 13 weeks onwards, and is well established by week 20. Antacid prophylaxis is warranted from 14 weeks, as would be RSI for elective surgery. Glycopyrrolate is a quaternary amide and too large to transfer across the placenta. Neostigmine, however, is transferred across the placenta and could lead to significant foetal bradycardia.

Nejdlova, M. and Johnson, T. (2012) Anaesthesia for non-obstetric procedures during pregnancy. *CEACCP*, **12(4):** 203–20.

SBA 51: answer = A – Seizure

The $sjVO_2$ is used to give an assessment of overall oxygenation and cerebral blood flow. The catheter is advanced into the jugular bulb and sits level with the C1/C2 disc. The $sjVO_2$ reflects the balance between oxygen supply and demand. Seizures will cause increased demand and the $sjVO_2$ will decrease. The other pathologies all reflect either a reduced demand or an increased oxygen delivery.

Elwishi, M. and Dinsmore, J. (2019) Monitoring the brain. *BJA Education*, **19(2):** 54–59.

SBA 52: answer = E – Change to a pressure-based trigger

An intra-aortic balloon pump has been placed post-operatively to support the coronary circulation and to increase cardiac output. Management of cardiac arrest following cardiac surgery utilises a modified BLS/ALS algorithm, as the underlying cause is often a post-operative arrhythmia. If the patient has a balloon pump *in situ* it is important that this is changed to a pressure-based trigger, as this will mean that it will continue to pump in combination with compressions if they are occurring at this stage. The IABP should not be turned off unless the patient is fully anticoagulated, and removal should only be done after discussion with a senior cardiologist or surgeon. Switching the ratio will not help in the immediate situation.

Brand, J., McDonald, A. and Dunning, J. (2018) Management of cardiac arrest following cardiac surgery. *BJA Education*, **18(1):** 16–22.

SBA 53: answer = A – Linear probe, 5–10MHz, 1–5cm depth

Ultrasound images are dependent on the probe used and the ultrasound frequency. Higher frequencies allow better resolution at shallower depths. Lower frequencies allow better images for deeper structures, but with a loss of spatial resolution. In this case, a curvilinear probe would be better suited to deeper nerves, as would a lower frequency. A depth of 1–5cm is appropriate to allow for inter-individual differences.

Carty, S. and Nicholls, B. (2007) Ultrasound-guided regional anaesthesia. *BJA Education*, **7(1):** 20–24.

SBA 54: answer = D – 2b

Evidence can be graded into four broad categories (some of which have subcategories), with '4' being the weakest evidence (expert opinion) and '1' being the strongest (systematic review or meta-analysis of randomised controlled trials). A well-designed cohort study falls into a 2b grading of evidence.

Smith, F., Tong, J. and Smith, J. (2006) Evidence-based medicine? *CEACCP*, **6(4):** 148–151.

SBA 55: answer = E – Joubert syndrome

Morquio syndrome and other mucopolysaccharidoses provide significant challenges for airway management. Of these, Hunter and Hurler syndromes are most challenging. Joubert syndrome is a cerebellar disorder and doesn't affect the airway and airway-related anatomy.

Raj, D. and Igor, L. (2015) Managing the difficult airway in a syndromic child. *BJA Education*, **15(1):** 7–14.

SBA 56: answer = D – Prevent hypothermia using warming devices

Hypothermia can cause vasoconstriction, reducing flap perfusion. This can occur frequently as the surgery is often prolonged (>8 hours) and large areas of the patient are exposed. Forced air warming devices can be used to prevent this. Using vasoconstrictors is a contentious subject. Although maintaining a mean arterial pressure close to the patient's normal is beneficial, vasoconstrictors may cause flap perforator vasoconstriction. Maintaining a haematocrit of 30–35% is most ideal, and excessive fluid therapy may cause flap oedema and failure. Therapeutic anticoagulation is not necessary, but prophylactic anticoagulation may be useful due to prolonged static periods.

Nimalan, N., Branford, O. and Stocks, G. (2015) Anaesthesia for free flap breast reconstruction. *BJA Education*, **(16)5:** 162–166.

SBA 57: answer = D – Cardiac defibrillation

Spinal cord stimulators are susceptible to being reprogrammed or to malfunction with electromagnetic interference. Therefore, they should be interrogated and turned off before surgery and procedures that induce EM interferences (including CT and MRI scans). At present, manufacturers advise against their use during pregnancy. The SCS should not be a barrier to defibrillation, or external pacing; however, it can be damaged by these processes.

Bull, C. and Baranidharan, G. (2020) Spinal cord stimulators and implications for anaesthesia. *BJA Education*, **20(6):** 182–183.

SBA 58: answer = B – Spirometry

Investigations should be targeted at assessing cardiac function – both electrical (ECG) and mechanical (echocardiogram) – and at detecting organ failure caused by hypoperfusion. Obstructive or restrictive lung defects (which would be detected by spirometry) are unusual, unless caused by concomitant pathology.

Nayak, S. and Booker, P. (2008) The Fontan circulation. *CEACCP*, **8(1):** 26–30.

SBA 59: answer = C – Bilirubin >3mg/dl

The King's College Criteria were designed to create a framework for referring centres to determine which patients are suitable for a liver transplant. There are minor variations in the referral criteria for patients who have had a paracetamol overdose and those who have acute liver failure of different aetiology. This specifically is the bilirubin level – which is not included in the overdose criteria.

Sharma, C. and Mehta, V. (2014) Paracetamol: mechanisms and updates. *CEACCP*, **14(4):** 153–158.

SBA 60: answer = B – Adrenaline

Follow the ALS cardiac arrest guidelines: although the patient remains in VF, there is no need for further doses of amiodarone. Therefore, the correct choice is adrenaline – which is given every 3–5 minutes. Lidocaine, magnesium and flecainide do not appear in the ALS algorithm.

Williams, S. and Bacon, R. (2017) Current recommendations on adult resuscitation. *BJA Education*, **17(3):** 99–104.

Practice Paper 3

CRQ 1: Tracheostomy

A patient on the intensive care unit is undergoing a semi-elective insertion of a percutaneous tracheostomy.

---

a What are the indications for a tracheostomy? (5 marks)

  i. ....

  ii. ....

  iii. ....

  iv. ....

  v. ....

b What are the possible consequences of insertion of a tracheostomy tube that is too short? (2 marks)

  i. ....

  ii. ....

c List 3 immediate, 3 early and 3 long-term complications of insertion of a percutaneous tracheostomy. (9 marks)

Immediate:

  i. ....

  ii. ....

  iii. ....

Early:

  i. ....

  ii. ....

  iii. ....

Long-term:

i. ....

ii. ....

iii. ....

The patient undergoes a successful percutaneous tracheostomy and is weaning well. Approximately 3 days after the procedure the patient develops respiratory distress and begins to desaturate. The bedside nurses have connected a Mapleson C system to the tracheostomy which is showing no movement of the bag and there is no $etCO_2$ showing on the monitor. The patient has a pulse.

d	Outline the initial management of the patient in respiratory distress with a tracheostomy.	(4 marks)

....

....

....

....

CRQ 2: Posterior fossa surgery

A 27-year-old man has been listed for surgery for an imaging-confirmed posterior fossa tumour. He has no other comorbidities and has had one previous anaesthetic for a knee arthroscopy in the past which was uneventful.

a   What structures are contained within the posterior fossa?   (3 marks)

i. ....

ii. ....

iii. ....

The neurosurgery team wish to perform the surgery in the sitting position and they mention that the patient is at risk of developing a venous air embolism.

b   List three other potential complications of the sitting position for neurosurgery (excluding venous air embolism).   (3 marks)

i. ....

ii. ....

iii. ....

c   During the procedure the surgical team wish to use intra-operative neuro-monitoring. List two adaptations to your anaesthetic technique to help facilitate this and avoid interference with monitoring.   (2 marks)

i. ....

ii. ....

d   Name three risk factors for the development of a venous air embolism, excluding patient positioning.   (3 marks)

i. ....

ii. ....

iii. ....

During the procedure there is a sudden drop in etCO$_2$ and the neurosurgeons state that there is air in the operating field. They suspect a venous air embolism.

e   List four steps in the management of a suspected venous air embolism.   (4 marks)

i. ....

ii. ....

iii. ....

iv. ....

The patient is stabilised and remains stable throughout the rest of the operation. The decision is made to extubate the patient following the procedure to establish neurological status.

f   Name three ways in which the risk of coughing on the endotracheal tube following the procedure can be minimised.   (3 marks)

i. ....

ii. ....

iii. ....

Posterior fossa syndrome can sometimes complicate the post-operative course in paediatric patients.

g   What is the defining feature of posterior fossa syndrome?   (1 mark)

....

h   Name one risk factor for the development of posterior fossa syndrome.   (1 mark)

....

CRQ 3: Eclampsia

A pregnant patient has presented to anaesthetic obstetric pre-operative clinic after being referred by the obstetricians. She is gravida 2 para 1 and her previous delivery was complicated by an eclamptic seizure and required a delivery under general anaesthetic. She has no other past medical history. The obstetricians are concerned about the possibility of her developing eclampsia again and would like the patient to have a pre-assessment appointment to discuss delivery options should the need arise.

| a | How is hypertension in pregnancy diagnosed? | (2 marks) |

....

....

| b | Explain the difference between chronic hypertension and gestational hypertension. | (1 mark) |

....

| c | Define pre-eclampsia. | (3 marks) |

....

....

....

| d | List five risk factors for the development of pre-eclampsia. | (5 marks) |

i. ....

ii. ....

iii. ....

iv. ....

v. ....

The obstetricians are considering starting some antihypertensive therapy to reduce the risk of premature delivery.

e List two antihypertensive therapies that the patient may be started on (with doses) to reduce the risk of premature delivery or maternal stroke. (2 marks)

i. ....

ii. ....

The patient presents at 36 weeks with tightening sensations across the abdomen. She has remained hypertensive and is beginning to show signs of severe pre-eclampsia.

f List three symptoms/signs that would suggest the patient now has severe pre-eclampsia (excluding blood pressure reading). (3 marks)

i. ....

ii. ....

iii. ....

g What is the first-line treatment for prevention of an eclamptic seizure? Include dose(s). (3 marks)

....

....

....

After treatment with antihypertensives the patient is stable but continues to have contractions. She wishes to have neuraxial blockade for her labour analgesia; however, the obstetricians have been concerned about the possibility of HELLP syndrome.

h Within what period of time should the most recent blood tests have been taken, prior to conducting the block? (1 mark)

....

CRQ 4:   Cardioplegia

A patient has been listed for a coronary artery bypass graft. The surgery is being performed on bypass and the surgeons will be using cardioplegia to facilitate the surgery.

a   List three reasons for the use of cardioplegia solution in bypass surgery.   (3 marks)

  i.   ....

  ii.   ....

  iii.   ....

b   Complete the following table of additives which are added to cardioplegia solution, and their associated physiological actions.   (8 marks)

Ion/solution added to cardioplegia	Physiological action
Potassium	Inactivates fast inward sodium channels and prevents myocyte action potential, thus invoking cardiac arrest

c What are the proposed benefits of using blood cardioplegia as opposed to crystalloid cardioplegia? (3 marks)

....

....

....

d List three complications of using cardioplegia during cardiac surgery. (3 marks)

i. ....

ii. ....

iii. ....

e For the following methods of cardioplegia administration, describe where the cannulae would be placed. (2 marks)

Anterograde: ....

Retrograde: ....

f Why is a transoesophageal echocardiogram important prior to the administration of cardioplegia? (1 mark)

....

CRQ 5: Back pain

You are asked to review a 45-year-old woman on the ward who has been admitted with severe lower back pain which is preventing mobilisation.

---

a Define chronic back pain. (2 marks)

....

....

b The patient is concerned that she has sciatica. List two symptoms or signs which would support this diagnosis. (2 marks)

i. ....

ii. ....

c List four risk factors for acute back pain progressing to chronic back pain. (4 marks)

i. ....

ii. ....

iii. ....

iv. ....

d List six "red flag" markers for serious spinal pathology in assessment of back pain. (6 marks)

i. ....

ii. ....

iii. ....

iv. ....

v. ....

vi. ....

e Assuming this patient has no other comorbidities, list two suitable pharmacological agents (with doses) which might form part of an initial management plan for lower back pain, according to NICE guidance. (2 marks)

i. ....

ii. ....

f Name four non-pharmacological strategies you could advise a patient for self-treatment of lower back pain. (4 marks)

i. ....

ii. ....

iii. ....

iv. ....

CRQ 6:   Pyloric stenosis

A 4-week-old male infant born at term weighing 5kg presents with projectile vomiting after feeds. He has been diagnosed with pyloric stenosis and is scheduled to undergo a pyloromyotomy. He is noted to have a heart rate of 160bpm, respiratory rate of 70/min and urine output of 5ml/hr. He is also noted to have a sunken anterior fontanelle and dry mucous membranes.

a   Estimate the percentage dehydration of this infant.   (1 mark)

....

b   What is the likely urgency of this surgical case (according to
        NCEPOD grading)?   (1 mark)

....

c   Describe, with doses/concentrations, an appropriate fluid regime
        for this patient.   (3 marks)

Resuscitation: ....

Maintenance: ....

....

d   Describe two mechanisms by which a hypokalaemia develops
        in patients with pyloric stenosis.   (2 marks)

  i.   ....

  ii. ....

e   Describe three strategies to reduce the risk of pulmonary aspiration
        of stomach contents during pyloromyotomy.   (3 marks)

  i.   ....

  ii. ....

  iii. ....

f Give two potential advantages of laparoscopic over open pyloromyotomy. (2 marks)

i. ....

ii. ....

g Describe an appropriate post-operative analgesia strategy for this patient. (2 marks)

....

....

h List six risk factors for post-operative apnoea in infants undergoing any surgery (not just pyloric stenosis). (6 marks)

i. ....

ii. ....

iii. ....

iv. ....

v. ....

vi. ....

CRQ 7: Cardiomyopathy in pregnancy

A 34-year-old woman, who has a background of cardiomyopathy, has been referred to obstetric pre-assessment clinic. She is gravida 2 para 1 and she is requesting a vaginal delivery.

a Define cardiomyopathy. (2 marks)

....

....

b Complete the following table of the types of cardiomyopathy. (9 marks)

Type of cardiomyopathy	Aetiology	Pathophysiology	Clinical features/ symptoms
Dilated			
Hypertrophic			
Restrictive			

The patient has an echocardiogram which is reported as having moderate–severe dilated cardiomyopathy with an ejection fraction of 30%.

c List four classes of medication that the patient may have been on prior to becoming pregnant. (2 marks)

i. .... & ....

ii. .... & ....

d What are the key broad anaesthetic goals in the peri-operative management of this patient? (4 marks)

....

....

....

....

e What would you advise this patient regarding her choice of anaesthetic / pain relief, and why? (3 marks)

....

....

....

CRQ 8: Neck trauma

A 25-year-old man has been brought to A&E from the local prison. He had been attacked by another prisoner who has used a home-made sharp object. On arrival he is complaining of neck swelling, difficulty breathing and change in voice. He is holding a large piece of blood-soaked gauze to his neck. The trauma team suspect he has sustained significant neck injury with damage to a major blood vessel and the ENT surgeon is worried about damage to the carotid artery or surrounding structures.

a List four main structures that lie within the carotid sheath. (4 marks)

i. ....

ii. ....

iii. ....

iv. ....

You opt to intubate the patient for airway protection and plan to take the patient to theatre for exploratory surgery. When the gauze is removed it is clear there is penetrating damage to the trachea as well as surrounding structures, and there is no obvious bleeding point. The patient is stable and cooperative.

b Which hard signs would prompt you to consider a diagnosis of aerodigestive tract injury? (4 marks)

i. ....

ii. ....

iii. ....

iv. ....

c List three ways in which the airway can be secured in this patient safely. (3 marks)

i. ....

ii. ....

iii. ....

d Assuming that the patient does not need cervical spine immobilisation, why is a blind bougie technique with direct laryngoscopy **not** appropriate in this patient? (2 marks)

....

....

e When placing the tracheal tube, how far should the cuff be advanced before connecting to a breathing circuit? (1 mark)

....

f List three other features of anaesthetic induction that should be *avoided* in patients with penetrating neck trauma. (3 marks)

i. ....

ii. ....

iii. ....

g If there was no evidence of penetrating injury but instead blunt neck trauma was suspected, list three red flag examination findings that would indicate the need for urgent airway intervention. (3 marks)

i. ....

ii. ....

iii. ....

CRQ 9: Breast surgery and flap reconstruction

A 54-year-old woman with breast cancer is scheduled for a total mastectomy and reconstruction. She has had chemotherapy prior to the surgery and the oncologists are happy that a reconstruction and mastectomy will be successful. She is an ex-smoker (gave up 3 weeks ago) and has been started recently on amlodipine for hypertension.

a What are the most common possible anatomical options for both pedicled and non-pedicled flaps for this patient? (3 marks)

Pedicled: ....

i. Non-pedicled (free flap): ....

ii. Non-pedicled (free flap): ....

b Describe the three main stages in free-flap reconstruction. (3 marks)

i. ....

ii. ....

iii. ....

c Outline the metabolic changes that the free flap undergoes in the first 5–10 minutes post its removal. (3 marks)

i. ....

ii. ....

iii. ....

The flap type the surgeons have chosen to use contains more skin than muscle.

d What is the oxygen consumption of the skin at rest in ml/min per 100g tissue? (1 mark)

....

e What are the possible issues specifically with flap reconstruction surgery that can be caused by cigarette smoking? (3 marks)

....

....

....

f List the key anaesthetic goals which will help prevent flap failure in the early and late period. (3 marks)

i. ....

ii. ....

iii. ....

The patient emerges from anaesthesia and is brought to HDU for post-operative flap monitoring.

g What features of the flap should nursing staff be checking to identify early flap failure? (4 marks)

i. ....

ii. ....

iii. ....

iv. ....

CRQ 10:   Critical incidents

A 31-year-old patient presents for a category 1 caesarean section. She has no medical history; this pregnancy has been uneventful and she has never had a general anaesthetic before. The rapid spinal is ineffective and conversion to GA is undertaken with suxamethonium, and propofol sevoflurane is used for maintenance of anaesthesia.

Five minutes post induction, the baby has been delivered, and you notice that the end tidal CO_2 is rising, the surgeon is asking for more relaxation, she is tachycardic and the temperature when taken is 38.7°C.

a	List four possible differential diagnoses.	(4 marks)

  i. ....

  ii. ....

 iii. ....

 iv. ....

b	You suspect a diagnosis of malignant hyperthermia. Outline the pathophysiology of this condition.	(6 marks)

....

....

....

....

....

....

c   Outline the clinical management in this case.   (8 marks)

....

....

....

....

....

....

....

....

d   The patient is admitted to intensive care following surgical closure and makes a full recovery. What two tests are needed going forward for the patient and close family?   (2 marks)

i.   ....

ii.   ....

CRQ 11: Ophthalmic surgery

A 93-year-old patient presents for cataract surgery. She is hypertensive and diabetic, dependent for all care.

a Label this diagram of the eye with the relevant anatomy that you will need to be aware of in order to safely proceed with your block of choice. (3 marks)

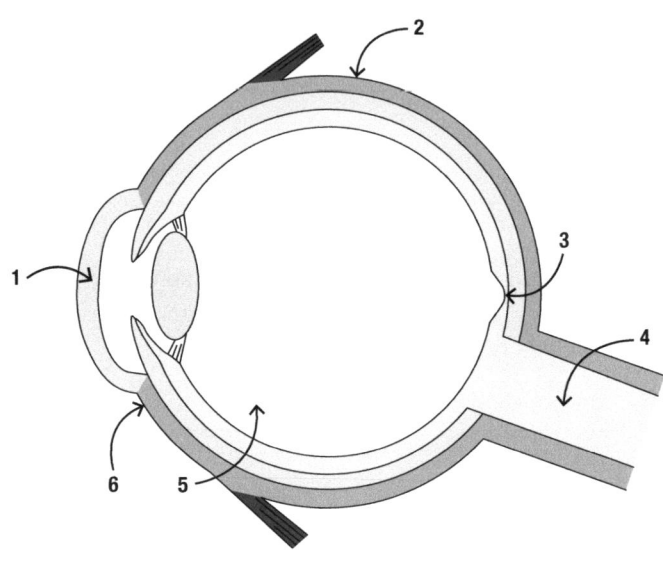

1. ....

2. ....

3. ....

4. ....

5. ....

6. ....

b Name the three most commonly performed blocks that may be used to facilitate this surgery, and state whether these are sharp or blunt needle techniques. (3 marks)

i. ....

ii. ....

iii. ....

c | What is normal intra-ocular pressure (IOP) and which three factors affect IOP? (4 marks)

Pressure: ....

i. **Factor:** ....

ii. **Factor:** ....

iii. **Factor:** ....

The nurse comes to inform you that the patient has had a cup of tea in the waiting room, that she is first on the list for this morning and is happy to have the procedure under block as long as she can have some mild sedation for anxiolysis.

d | (i) Can the list go ahead as planned? (ii) Why/why not? (2 marks)

i. ....

ii. ....

e | You perform your block of choice, and whilst compressing the globe the patient loses consciousness. Describe the neurogenic mechanism for the oculo-cardiac reflex. (6 marks)

Cause: ....

....

Afferent pathway: ....

....

Efferent pathway: ....

....

f | You greet the next patient and on taking the history you realise that this patient is unsuitable for regional block. List four reasons why this might be the case. (2 marks)

i. .... & ....

ii. .... & ....

CRQ 12: Head and neck cancer

A 58-year-old man presents for resection of a laryngeal tumour which becomes periodically obstructive and has gradually become worse over the course of the last few months.

a What are the risk factors for development of head and neck cancers? (3 marks)

i. ....

ii. ....

iii. ....

b What patient, environmental and anaesthetic implications are there for managing this patient? (5 marks)

i. **Patient:** ....

ii. **Patient:** ....

i. **Environmental:** ....

ii. **Environmental:** ....

Anaesthetic: ....

c The patient is booked for a panendoscopy. The surgeon requires a clear view; she has asked which technique you will use. Please outline one advantage (A) and three disadvantages (D) of these ventilation strategies for panendoscopy.

(6 marks)

	MLT and IPPV	Supraglottic jet	Subglottic jet
A	....	....	....
D	....	....	....
	....	....	....
	....	....	....

d Post-operatively there is marked swelling and the surgeon is unsure whether the airway will remain patent after ventilation ceases. What are the options in this case? (2 marks)

i. ....

ii. ....

e What post-operative considerations would you have for this patient? (4 marks)

....

....

....

....

SBA 1:

You have anaesthetised a 72-year-old woman undergoing laser debulking of a laryngeal tumour. You are alerted by the surgeon to evidence of an airway fire. The surgeon has stepped away and stopped using the laser.

What is the next appropriate step?

A. Douse the operating field with water
B. Perform urgent bronchoscopy
C. Remove the laser endotracheal tube
D. Stop ventilation
E. Disconnect the O_2 source/piping

SBA 2:

A 60-year-old man with a history of heavy smoking and alcohol misuse attends the pre-operative assessment clinic prior to major head and neck cancer surgery.

Which of the following are contraindications to free flap formation?

A. Factor V Leiden
B. Sickle cell disease
C. Previous flap failure
D. Well-controlled polycythaemia rubra vera
E. Renal failure

SBA 3:

A 46-year-old woman is being considered for surgical management of her trigeminal neuralgia. She has found no benefit from pharmacotherapy and psychosocial support.

Which of the following is most likely to provide good long-term (>10 years) pain relief?

A. Neurectomy at Gasserian ganglion
B. Microvascular decompression
C. Laser neurolysis of distal ganglion branches
D. Chemical ablation of Gasserian ganglion
E. Terminal nerve branch blockade and ablation

SBA 4:

A baby is delivered at 36 weeks via an uncomplicated caesarean section for failure to progress. The baby was taken immediately to the Resuscitaire by the delivery midwife. The baby has blue extremities, a heart rate of 120bpm, is active and has a prompt response to stimulation, but has a slow and irregular respiration rate.

What is the baby's APGAR score?

A. 5
B. 6
C. 7
D. 8
E. 9

SBA 5:

A 64-year-old man with COPD has presented acutely short of breath to A&E. He has been progressively short of breath on exertion and has now developed peripheral oedema. On examination he has a raised JVP and a right ventricular heave. A transthoracic echo is performed which shows an estimated systolic pulmonary artery pressure of 40mmHg.

In order to exclude thromboembolic disease as a cause, what is the most sensitive method of excluding clot?

A. Transthoracic echocardiography
B. Transoesophageal echocardiography
C. CT pulmonary angiogram (CTPA)
D. Right-heart catheterisation
E. Isotope perfusion scanning

SBA 6:

A 72-year-old man is reviewed in the pre-operative assessment clinic before his transurethral resection of bladder tumour (TURBT). He has an ECG which shows progressive lengthening of the PR interval followed by the failed conduction of an atrial beat. He is asymptomatic and his exercise tolerance is normal.

What is the correct pre-operative intervention/investigation required for this patient?

A. Permanent pacemaker insertion
B. No intervention required
C. Pre-operative angiogram
D. Echocardiogram
E. CPEX testing

SBA 7:

A 26-year-old primigravida has had an epidural sited for labour analgesia. Following the first test dose of 20ml low dose mix (levobupivacaine 0.125% and fentanyl 2mcg/ml) she develops dizziness, peri-orbital tingling and intermittent loss of consciousness.

What is the most beneficial treatment for this reaction?

A. 1.5ml/kg of 20% lipid emulsion (Intralipid) bolus followed by an infusion of 15ml/kg/hour
B. 2g $MgSO_4$ stat followed by a magnesium infusion
C. Intubation and ventilation with propofol as induction agent
D. Start CPR
E. Place the patient in the left lateral position

SBA 8:

A 30-year-old primigravida has presented in labour at 37 weeks with the foetus in breech position. There has been one episode of foetal bradycardia which has recovered. She has moderate aortic stenosis and was booked for an elective caesarean section at 38 weeks. The obstetricians suggest she requires a category 2 caesarean section rather than allowing the labour to proceed.

What is the best anaesthetic technique to facilitate safe delivery?

A. General anaesthetic with fentanyl and propofol
B. Spinal with heavy bupivacaine
C. CSE with low dose spinal
D. Epidural
E. General anaesthetic with fentanyl, ketamine and rocuronium

SBA 9:

A 32-year-old woman has presented for posterior fossa surgery in the sitting position. The operating surgeon feels that this surgery is particularly high risk for the development of a venous air embolism (VAE).

Which of the following is the most sensitive intra-operative marker to detect a VAE?

A. $etCO_2$
B. Mean arterial pressure
C. Jugular bulb saturation
D. Near infra-red spectroscopy
E. Transthoracic Doppler

SBA 10:

A 65-year-old patient with a 14-year history of heart transplantation is due to undergo an elective total hip arthroplasty.

Which of the following drugs is unlikely to have any direct effect on either chronotropy or inotropy of the transplanted heart?

A. Atropine
B. Isoprenaline
C. Adrenaline
D. Dobutamine
E. Dopamine

SBA 11:

A 43-year-old patient presents for a trapeziectomy under axillary block with sedation.

Which of the following is not an element of the 'stop before you block' process?

A. Must only be initiated by the anaesthetist performing the block
B. Must be completed immediately prior to needle insertion
C. The surgical site marking should be checked
D. The site and side of the block should be checked with the patient and consent form
E. This should be a separate process to the WHO checklist

SBA 12:

Which of the following is not a ligament involved in the stabilisation of the spine?

A. Interspinous ligament
B. Posterior longitudinal ligament
C. Ligamentum flavum
D. Transverse spinous ligament
E. Anterior longitudinal ligament

SBA 13:

You respond to an emergency buzzer in a labour room in the delivery suite. A 39-week pregnant 33-year-old woman (G3P1) has collapsed and CPR has been commenced. You have rapidly secured the airway, commenced ventilation and a midwife is providing manual uterine displacement. After 4 minutes of CPR, the rhythm is noted to be pulseless electrical activity (PEA).

What would be the next most important step?

A. Atropine 600mcg IV bolus
B. Resuscitative hysterotomy
C. 120J biphasic defibrillation
D. 900mg IV amiodarone
E. 1.2g IV magnesium infusion

SBA 14:

A 46-year-old man is anaesthetised for a craniotomy and resection of tumour. A neurophysiologist is in attendance and has applied full electroencephalography (EEG) monitoring. You deliver an intravenous induction with propofol and maintain anaesthesia with 1.0 MAC sevoflurane.

Compared to the pre-induction baseline, which of the following EEG changes is most likely after 1 hour of sevoflurane maintenance anaesthesia?

A. Burst suppression
B. Decreased alpha wave power
C. Increased beta wave power
D. Decreased delta wave power
E. Increased theta wave power

SBA 15:

A 68-year-old woman has presented to the pre-operative assessment clinic for a CPEX test. She has been listed for a pneumonectomy for an underlying lung malignancy.

Below which peak oxygen consumption (VO_2 peak) is considered a contraindication to pneumonectomy surgery?

A. 10ml O_2/kg/min
B. 12ml O_2/kg/min
C. 15ml O_2/kg/min
D. 17ml O_2/kg/min
E. 20ml O_2/kg/min

SBA 16:

An 8-week pregnant, 28-year-old woman with long-standing T1DM is listed for a trapeziectomy and grafting, under the plastic surgery team. She has evidence of peripheral neuropathy affecting her lower limbs up to her ankles, diabetic retinopathy, and controls her blood sugars with a basal-bolus insulin regimen. You decide to perform a supraclavicular block.

Which of the following perineural adjuncts is most appropriate to extend block duration?

A. Adrenaline
B. Dexmedetomidine
C. Dexamethasone
D. Magnesium
E. Diclofenac sodium

SBA 17:

At what level do the vagal trunks descend through the diaphragm?

A. T8
B. T10
C. T12
D. L1
E. L2

SBA 18:

You are anaesthetising a 22-year-old man for surgical excision of a right ear cholesteatoma. During the procedure, the surgeon suggests that the surgical field is obscured by bleeding.

Which of the following is not a suitable method of optimising the operative field?

A. Reducing PEEP from 5cmH$_2$O to 1cmH$_2$O
B. Aiming for an arterial PCO$_2$ of 4–5kPa
C. Adjusting the patient to 10 degrees Trendelenburg
D. Minimising the inspiratory time during controlled ventilation
E. 50mg/kg IV magnesium bolus over 5 minutes

SBA 19:

You are due to anaesthetise a 74-year-old man for a carotid endarterectomy. He had a transient ischaemic attack 36 hours prior, causing right hemiparesis, amaurosis fugax and left-sided facial signs. His medical history includes atrial fibrillation, hypertension, coronary heart disease (with a single LAD stent) and type 2 diabetes.

Which of the following medications would you stop pre-operatively?

A. Clopidogrel 75mg OD
B. Aspirin 75mg OD
C. Bisoprolol 2.5mg OD
D. Ramipril 1.25mg ON
E. Metformin 500mg BD

SBA 20:

Which of the following surgical procedures most commonly results in chronic post-surgical pain?

A. Amputation
B. Thoracotomy
C. Mastectomy
D. Inguinal hernia repair
E. Sternotomy

SBA 21:

An otherwise well 2-year-old child presents to A&E following 2 days of diarrhoea and vomiting. On clinical examination, the child appears irritable, with slightly sunken eyes. He has warm extremities and dry mucous membranes. His vital signs are as follows: pulse 135bpm, blood pressure 95/60mmHg, respiratory rate 32, oxygen saturation 98% on room air. Capillary refill time was 3 seconds.

What is the estimated percentage of dehydration for this child?

A. 0–2%
B. 3–5%
C. 6–9%
D. 10–12%
E. 13–15%

SBA 22:

A 24-year-old woman presented with increased confusion and aggression and so has been sedated in A&E. She is noted to have photophobia and neck stiffness. Her housemate reports that she had a recent cough, but this has settled. A capillary blood glucose was performed which was 6.7mmol/L. A lumbar puncture was performed and yielded the following result:

White cell count: 56/mm³ (80% lymphocytes) (0–8)
Red cell count: 1/mm³ (0–5)
Glucose: 4.2mmol/L (2.8–4.2)
Protein: 0.78g/L (0.15–0.45)

What is the most likely diagnosis?

A. Viral meningitis
B. Bacterial meningitis
C. HIV encephalitis
D. Toxoplasmosis
E. Normal CSF result

SBA 23:

A 74-year-old man presents following a fall secondary to myocardial infarction. A pelvic X-ray performed the following day – due to increased hip pain – showed a fractured neck of femur. In addition to this he was commenced on ticagrelor in A&E for the MI.

At what point after receiving ticagrelor would it be acceptable to perform a neuraxial block for correction of his neck of femur fracture?

A. 24 hours
B. 72 hours
C. 5 days
D. 7 days
E. 14 days

SBA 24:

Which of the following statements is incorrect with regard to malignant hyperthermia?

A. Prophylactic dantrolene is not recommended for use in susceptible individuals
B. Activated charcoal filters can be added to both the inspiratory and expiratory limb of the anaesthetic machine to bind volatile anaesthetic agents
C. Anti-parkinsonian medication should be continued in the peri-operative period to avoid the possibility of neuroleptic malignant syndrome
D. Patients with malignant hyperthermia are at increased risk of serotonin syndrome
E. TIVA can be used safely in patients with malignant hyperthermia

SBA 25:

A woman presents in labour at 5cm dilation with a history of von Willebrand disease and resultant abnormal coagulation. She wants a remifentanil PCA, having discussed this in the obstetric clinic.

Which of the following statements is not accurate?

A. Remifentanil PCA is not as effective as epidural analgesia
B. Remifentanil is unlicensed for this indication
C. The context-sensitive half-time is 5 minutes
D. Remifentanil rapidly crosses the placenta due to high lipophilicity
E. APGAR scores do not differ significantly between remifentanil PCA and epidural analgesia

SBA 26:

A 75-year-old patient has presented to the pre-operative assessment clinic ahead of his posterior fossa tumour removal.

Which of the following co-morbidities is an **absolute** contraindication for posterior fossa surgery in the sitting position?

A. Ventriculo-atrial shunt
B. Severe autonomic neuropathy
C. Patent foramen ovale
D. Uncontrolled hypertension
E. Rheumatoid arthritis affecting the neck

SBA 27:

A 58-year-old woman with a tissue mitral valve replacement is due to undergo multiple dental extractions under general anaesthesia.

What is the correct choice of antibiotic for this patient for the prophylaxis of infective endocarditis?

A. Meropenem
B. Co-amoxiclav
C. Ciprofloxacin
D. Clarithromycin
E. No prophylaxis needed

SBA 28:

A patient on long-term anticoagulation is scheduled for a left total hip replacement after a traumatic fall.

Which of the following options correctly identifies the acceptable time after drug administration for central neuraxial blockade performance?

A. 30 minutes after unfractionated heparin
B. 5 days after clopidogrel
C. 8 hours after tirofiban
D. 3 days after ticagrelor
E. 36 hours after abciximab

SBA 29:

Which of the following nerves is responsible for tensing the vocal cords and aiding in phonation?

A. Recurrent laryngeal nerve
B. Posterior laryngeal nerve
C. Inferior laryngeal nerve
D. Superior laryngeal nerve
E. Trigeminal nerve

SBA 30:

A 47-year-old female complains of a newly hoarse voice following a laparoscopic cholecystectomy one day prior. She has a background of obesity and obstructive sleep apnoea, and her airway was managed with a size 7.5 cuffed Mallinckrodt endotracheal tube during the general anaesthetic. On performance of a flexible nasal endoscopy (FNE) by the ENT team, her right vocal cord is noted to be in the para-median position.

Which of the following best explains the reason for this?

A. Unopposed action of the right vocalis muscle
B. Right phrenic nerve injury
C. Damage to the right recurrent lingual nerve
D. Unopposed action of the right cricothyroid muscle
E. Loss of tone in right cricoarytenoid muscle

SBA 31:

You review a 26-year-old man brought into A&E after being extracted unconscious from a burning vinyl factory. He was intubated on the scene by the helicopter emergency medical service (HEMS), due to being unrousable, hypoxic and hypotensive. At present, he has a heart rate of 56bpm, O_2 saturation 90% with an FiO_2 of 1.0, BP of 106/72mmHg supported with 9ml/hr 1mg/ml metaraminol infusion, and is mechanically ventilated. He has a serum lactate of 8.7mmol/L, PaO_2 9.2kPa, PCO_2 8.4kPa, and pH 7.1. His pupils are fixed and unreactive. What is the most likely cause?

A. Brainstem death
B. Cyanide poisoning
C. Alveolar deposits of aldehydes
D. Carbon monoxide poisoning
E. Methaemoglobin

SBA 32:

A 57-year-old man with a history of advanced pancreatic cancer has been admitted following an ischaemic stroke. He is currently nil by mouth due to unsafe swallow, and the stroke team are concerned about opioid withdrawal, as he was previously on 160mg of morphine sulfate (MST) modified release BD.

Please choose the correct IV conversion that the patient should be commenced on.

A. Background: 5mg/hr. Bolus: 2mg
B. Background: 3mg/hr. Bolus: 1.5mg
C. Background: 6mg/hr. Bolus: 2mg
D. Background: 3mg/hr. Bolus: 3mg
E. Background: 6mg/hr. Bolus: 1mg

SBA 33:

Which of the following is least likely to cause haemodynamic instability in a patient with a Fontan circulation?

A. Using metaraminol
B. Arrhythmias
C. Hypercarbia
D. Hypovolaemia
E. Laparoscopic surgery

SBA 34:

A 74-year-old man, with a previous history of T2DM and asthma, has been intubated and ventilated for T1RF secondary to acute respiratory distress syndrome (ARDS).

Which of the following is not an indication for the use of airway pressure release ventilation (APRV)?

A. Sepsis
B. Restrictive lung disease
C. Failure of 'trial of proning'
D. Obesity
E. Failure of 'low tidal volume ventilation'

SBA 35:

An 89-year-old man was anaemic post-operatively following an emergency neck of femur repair. He was transfused 3 units of cross-matched packed red cells, and 5 hours later on the orthopaedic ward he became acutely short of breath and febrile. A subsequent chest X-ray showed bilateral pulmonary infiltrates.

What is the most likely cause of his acute shortness of breath?

A. Transfusion-related acute lung injury (TRALI)
B. Transfusion-related circulatory overload (TACO)
C. Transfusion of non-ABO compatible blood
D. Transfusion-associated graft-versus-host disease (GvHD)
E. Non-haemolytic febrile blood reaction

SBA 36:

A 19-year-old patient with a history of Hodgkin's lymphoma has been listed for an elective splenectomy. He is not currently receiving immunosuppressive therapy.

With regard to peri-operative vaccination (pneumococcal, Hib, meningococcal and influenza), which of the following is correct?

A. Elective splenectomy patients do not need vaccinations peri-operatively
B. Vaccinations should be given 14 days prior to splenectomy
C. Vaccinations should be given 7 days prior to splenectomy
D. Vaccinations should be given 14 days post-operatively
E. Vaccinations should be given 3 months post-operatively

SBA 37:

You are consenting a 36-year-old woman in the delivery suite for an epidural.

Which of the following is not a validated recommendation for safe insertion of epidurals for labour analgesia?

A. 2% chlorhexidine gluconate in 10% alcohol spray to skin, air dried
B. Tunnelled epidural catheters
C. The use of non-Luer lock epidural connections
D. Antibiotic prophylaxis
E. Prophylactic low molecular weight heparin can be given 4 hours after insertion

SBA 38:

An arterial line has been inserted for a prolonged neurosurgical procedure in the sitting position.

At which level should the arterial transducer be placed?

A. Level with the heart
B. Level with the shoulder
C. Level with the temple
D. Level with the external auditory meatus
E. Level with the operating table

SBA 39:

Which of the following conditions is not an indication for cardiac transplantation?

A. Advanced heart failure (NYHA III/IV) with recurrent admissions despite maximal medical therapy
B. Recurrent life-threatening ventricular arrhythmia despite ICD
C. Acute cardiogenic shock requiring infusion of inotropic agents
D. Refractory angina without further therapeutic options
E. Severe ventricular aneurysm with thrombus formation

SBA 40:

A 32-year-old woman has been listed for acromioclavicular joint exploration and repair, following an injury whilst cycling 8 months prior. You have performed an interscalene block (ISB) to facilitate the shoulder surgery.

Which of the following is the most common complication following an ISB?

A. Phrenic nerve palsy
B. Horner's syndrome
C. Intrathecal drug administration
D. Local anaesthetic toxicity
E. Hypotension

SBA 41:

When considering the physiological changes of pregnancy, which of the following is incorrect?

A. Oxygen requirement increases by 60% during pregnancy
B. Progesterone causes a lowering of the response threshold for CO_2 in the respiratory centre
C. ALP (alkaline phosphatase) may be increased in the third trimester
D. Plasma cholinesterase activity increases from the 10th week of pregnancy
E. FRC (functional residual capacity) is decreased by 30% in the supine position

SBA 42:

You are anaesthetising a 61kg, 43-year-old woman for orthognathic surgery. She has no significant medical problems and is not on any regular medication. Her airway assessment pre-operatively is as follows: mouth opening 4cm, Mallampati score 2, jaw protrusion grade A, full range of motion of neck.

What would be the most appropriate airway intervention for this procedure?

A. Laryngeal mask airway – size 4
B. Microlaryngoscopy tube – size 6
C. Mallinckrodt endotracheal tube – size 7
D. Nasal intubation – size 7
E. South facing RAE tube – size 7

SBA 43:

You are anaesthetising a 64-year-old woman for examination under anaesthesia and measurement of intra-ocular pressure.

Which of the following is known to raise intra-ocular pressure?

A. Atropine
B. Sub-Tenon's block
C. Peribulbar block
D. Reverse Trendelenburg position
E. Diclofenac sodium

SBA 44:

Which of the following drugs which act on the endocannabinoid system has been licensed in the UK for treatment of pain?

A. Nabiximols (Sativex)
B. Nabilone
C. Epidiolex (cannabidiol)
D. Dronabinol
E. Vapourised THC

SBA 45:

With regard to the provision of day case surgery in the NHS, which of the following statements is incorrect regarding safe operating policy as per RCoA guidance?

A. Morbidly obese patients can be managed in a day case surgery environment
B. Ex-premature infants can be managed in the day case surgery unit provided they are >60 weeks post conceptual age
C. Emergency procedures can be done as part of a day case surgery list
D. There is no upper limit to patient age for day surgery
E. There must be an inpatient paediatric facility within the same hospital site if a paediatric list is offered

SBA 46:

A 24-year-old patient has been admitted to the resus department with diabetic ketoacidosis and urinary tract infection. The patient has been started on IV fluids, antibiotics, and a fixed rate insulin infusion which is currently running at 0.1 units/kg/hour. The A&E team have asked for an ICU review as they are concerned that the patient does not seem to be improving.

In which of the following situations would the rate of the FRII need to be increased?

A. Blood ketone concentration has reduced by 0.6mmol/L in an hour
B. Venous bicarbonate has increased by 3mmol/L in an hour
C. Venous bicarbonate has increased by 2mmol/L in an hour
D. Capillary blood glucose has reduced by 3mmol/L in an hour
E. Capillary blood glucose has reduced by 5mmol/L in an hour

SBA 47:

A 26-year-old woman presents to day surgery for a knee arthroscopy in the day surgery unit. She is first on the list and is expecting to go home in the afternoon. She has had severe PONV after every general anaesthetic and has consented to the procedure being performed under spinal anaesthesia.

What would be the optimal choice of intrathecal anaesthesia?

A. 0.5% hyperbaric bupivacaine with fentanyl
B. 0.5% hyperbaric bupivacaine with preservative-free morphine
C. 0.5% hyperbaric bupivacaine
D. 2% hyperbaric prilocaine with fentanyl
E. 2% hyperbaric prilocaine

SBA 48:

When considering medical devices that are attached to patients, Type B electrical equipment is limited to which of the following leakage currents?

A. <1µA
B. ≤10µA
C. ≤100µA
D. ≤10mA
E. ≤100mA

SBA 49:

Which of the following is true regarding amniotic fluid embolism (AFE)?

A. AFE occurs in three phases; phase 3 is characterised by disseminated intravascular coagulation
B. Foetal distress is a rare sign of an AFE
C. Tranexamic acid should not be given until thromboelastography has been performed
D. Serum complement levels are diagnostic in AFE
E. Hypofibrinogenaemia is a common finding

SBA 50:

A 23-year-old man has presented to A&E following a road traffic accident. The patient was not wearing a seatbelt and his head struck the windscreen of the car. He was transported with a GCS of 6, and has been intubated in A&E by the anaesthetic team.

Which of the following is not part of the key management goals for a patient with traumatic brain injury?

A. Early instigation of sedation/barbiturate coma
B. Aim $PaCO_2$ 4.5–5.0 kPa
C. Aim blood glucose 6–10mmol/L
D. Maintain PaO_2 >11kPa
E. Early administration of steroids

SBA 51:

A 58-year-old woman is due to undergo a mastectomy and axillary node clearance for breast cancer. She has a history of hypertension, psoriasis and chronic chest wall pain secondary to previous radiation therapy – for which she takes regular morphine. Your consultant decides to place a unilateral paravertebral catheter for analgesia in this patient.

What marks the anterior border of the paravertebral space?

A. Parietal pleura
B. Thoracic vertebrae
C. Head of ribs
D. Visceral pleura
E. Sympathetic chain

SBA 52:

A 72-year-old smoker has been admitted to hospital with a worsening cough and breathlessness. She is mildly confused, and on examination, she is cachectic with no other positive findings. Her sodium is 107mmol/L, potassium 4.5mmol/L, urea 4.8mmol/L and creatinine is 70μmol/L. Serum osmolality is 260mOsm/kg and urine osmolality is 240mOsm/kg. Urinary sodium is 40mmol/L.

What is the most appropriate first-line management plan for this patient?

A. Fluid restriction
B. Desmopressin
C. Demeclocycline
D. Tolvaptan
E. Hypertonic saline

SBA 53:

You have been asked to review a 58-year-old woman in A&E for consideration of intubation. She has recently been reviewed by her dentist and commenced on co-amoxiclav for a dental abscess. She has not been reviewed by a GP.

Which of the following symptoms is most suggestive of imminent airway compromise?

A. Stridor
B. Dysphagia
C. Lack of tongue protrusion
D. Odynophagia
E. Trismus

SBA 54:

A 61-year-old woman has presented in the pre-operative assessment clinic prior to a lower limb revascularisation procedure. She has severe calf claudication when mobilising, and moderate ischaemic limb pain at rest. She currently takes amitriptyline 75mg daily and gabapentin 300mg twice daily for her pain.

Which of the following analgesics should be avoided for limb revascularisation surgery?

A. Amitriptyline
B. Gabapentin
C. Prilocaine
D. Tramadol
E. Diclofenac sodium

SBA 55:

You are due to anaesthetise a 73-year-old man for a video-assisted thoracoscopic surgery (VATS) left lung segmentectomy. As part of your pain relief strategy, you plan a paravertebral block.

What ligament is pierced to enter the paravertebral space during injection?

A. Anterior longitudinal
B. Superior costotransverse
C. Supraspinous
D. Paravertebral
E. Intertransverse

SBA 56:

A 15-year-old girl has presented to day surgery for an elective adenotonsillectomy following multiple bouts of tonsillitis over the last 2 years, with a significant time off school. She is now refusing to have surgery and refusing any pre-admission observations, stating that she never agreed to having the surgery. Her mother is adamant she did want the surgery and wants to continue, having signed the consent form in clinic, and being unable to return to the hospital at a later time due to work commitments.

What is the safest way to proceed with this patient?

A. Cancel the patient and re-book at a later date
B. Proceed with the surgery but offer oral midazolam sedation
C. Place the patient at the end of the list to give the patient more time to consider surgery
D. Continue with surgery
E. Contact Trust lawyer

SBA 57:

A 23-year-old man is brought to A&E by ambulance. He collapsed while taking part in a triathlon on a particularly hot day. He has been found to have a rectal temperature of 40.8°C and is being treated for heatstroke.

Which of the following treatments is best in the initial management of exertional heatstroke?

A. Cold water immersion
B. Paracetamol
C. Dantrolene
D. 0.9% sodium chloride with 40mmol/L potassium chloride
E. Cold saline body cavity lavage

SBA 58:

A 21-year-old patient presents for an emergency laparoscopic salpingectomy. She is an ex-smoker and now vapes heavily.

Which of the following statements concerning vaping is true?

A. Vaping devices have not been known to cause burns
B. There are currently three generations of vaping devices
C. Cannabinoids are a legal additive in the UK
D. Vaping has no effect on platelet function
E. Acetone, silicates and metallic contamination are not found in inhaled vapour

SBA 59:

A 56-year-old woman has undergone a laparoscopic hysterectomy in a steep head-down position. Following the procedure she has weakness when abducting her shoulder, and paraesthesia across the lateral shoulder aspect and arm.

What is the most likely part of the brachial plexus that has been injured?

A. C5/C6 nerve root
B. Superior trunk
C. Middle trunk
D. Inferior trunk
E. Lateral cord

SBA 60:

You are called to review a 72-year-old post-operative patient, as the recovery nurse is concerned they remain in severe pain. The patient had an elective functional endoscopic sinus surgery (FESS) and has already required 10mg of IV morphine.

Which of the following is not a reliable method to assess pain scores?

A. The Pain in Advanced Dementia (PAINAD) tool
B. Cardiorespiratory parameters
C. Behaviour pain scale
D. Opiate consumption
E. Doloplus-2 tool

CRQ 1: answer guidance

Syllabus	CT_IS_07, AM_IK_04, AM_IK_06
Question type	Easy: pass mark 14
Topic	**Tracheostomy management**
Aim	To be able to correctly identify the indications and possible complications after insertion of a tracheostomy.
Pass requirements	Recall the management of the obstructed tracheostomy.

Q	Answer	Marks	Guidance
a	• Prolonged mechanical ventilation • Pulmonary toilet • Airway protection • As part of a surgical procedure • Upper airway obstruction	5	1 mark per correct answer. The most common indication on the ICU is to facilitate weaning of respiratory support.
b	• The tip of the tube may impinge on the posterior tracheal wall • The tip of the tube may sit in the subcutaneous tissue • The tube cuff may herniate upwards into superior larynx and vocal cords • The tube can become displaced and cause decannulation	2	1 mark per correct answer. Each of these may eventually cause loss of airway, critical hypoxia and cardiac arrest.
c	**Immediate:** aspiration, haemorrhage, air embolism, failure, structural damage to tracheal rings	3	Loss of airway can happen at any time so can only count as one mark within the question.
	Early: delayed haemorrhage, tube displacement, surgical emphysema, pneumomediastinum, pneumothorax, infection, tracheal necrosis, tracheo-arterial fistula, trachea-oesophageal fistula, dysphagia	3	
	Long-term: tracheal stenosis, decannulation, tracheocutaneous fistula, scar	3	
d	• Remove speaking valve/cap/inner tube	1	This must be in the correct order as there is an algorithm to follow. There is no point removing the tracheostomy before attempting other manoeuvres. The exception is deflating the cuff, as this could be done first.
	• Attempt to pass suction catheter	1	
	• Deflate cuff	1	
	• Remove tracheostomy tube	1	

Insertion of a percutaneous tracheostomy is one of the most common procedures in the intensive care setting and is commonly performed by anaesthetists and intensivists; thus it is important to be aware of the complications of their insertion. Furthermore it is essential to be able to competently manage the blocked tracheostomy. There is a national safety guideline on the management of the blocked tracheostomy that should be placed at the bed-space of every patient with a tracheostomy. It is important to remember that this changes if the patient has had a laryngectomy or other upper airway procedure.

Lewith, H. and Athanassoglou, V. (2019) Update on management of tracheostomy. *BJA Education*, **19(11):** 370–376.

National Tracheostomy Safety Project. *Cuff management*. Available at: www.tracheostomy.org. uk/storage/files/Cuff%20management.pdf (accessed 9 February 2022).

CRQ 2: answer guidance

Syllabus	NA_IK_09, NA_IS_06
Question type	Medium: pass mark 12
Topic	**Posterior fossa surgery**
Aim	To understand the basic considerations for posterior fossa surgery, including patient position and the risks involved, as well as specific management of neurosurgical emergencies.
Pass requirements	Knowledge of management of acute venous air embolism during posterior fossa surgery.

Q	Answer	Marks	Guidance
a	• Brainstem • Cerebellum • Lower cranial nerves (cranial nerves 7–12) • Sigmoid/transverse/occipital sinus (dural venous sinuses) • Cerebral aqueduct	3	1 mark per correct answer. Not enough if candidate mentions only one cranial nerve; must mention a range of nerves or group them as 'lower' to score one mark.
b	• Cardiovascular instability due to venous pooling, as well as variable cardiovascular response in older patients • Pneumocephalus • Macroglossia leading to airway compromise and post-operative airway obstruction • Quadriplegia (due to prolonged focal pressure on cord)	3	1 mark per correct answer. Other cardiovascular responses could be dramatic hypo-/hypertension or development of peri-operative arrhythmias. One mark for cardiovascular responses in total.

Q	Answer	Marks	Guidance
c	• Maintain constant levels of anaesthetic agent to prevent acute changes in monitoring response • Avoidance of neuromuscular blockers • Use of total intravenous anaesthesia	2	1 mark per correct answer. Although it is assumed TIVA and maintaining constant levels are similar, they are each worth a mark as it is possible to undertake SSEP/MEP under volatile anaesthesia, providing neurophysiologists are aware at beginning of the procedure and there are no dramatic changes in volatile concentration.
d	• Hypovolaemia (low venous pressure) • Large surface area open to air • Long procedure time • Mayfield pins	3	1 mark per correct answer.
e	• Flood surgical site with saline or saline-soaked swabs • Lower surgical site to below right atrium (head-downward tilt) • Aspirate air from central line • Place patient in left lateral (Durant) position • Jugular venous compression	4	1 mark per correct answer. Use of PEEP can be combined with lowering the surgical site; however, on its own it does not form part of the initial management.
f	• Use of opiate to suppress the coughing reflex (use of remifentanil as TIVA technique or single bolus opiate) • Deep extubation following spontaneous breathing being established • Exchange ETT for supraglottic airway device • Use of lidocaine spray around cords or bolus IV	3	1 mark per correct answer. This is normally achieved using remifentanil, but other methods are also acceptable.
g	Temporary and complete loss of speech after posterior fossa surgery	1	This can last for a number of months but is usually self-limiting.
h	• Medulloblastoma-type tumours • Midline location of tumour	1	

Posterior fossa surgery is mostly performed in children; however, it is common in neurosurgical centres to perform this type of surgery on a wide range of patients. Commonly venous air embolism has been considered a major risk; however, there are other risks such as concealed haemorrhage and damage to neurological structures. Although not all cases need neuro-monitoring such as SSEP or MEP, it is important to understand which common practices can affect these, such as changing volatile concentration or neuromuscular blockade. This is a common topic in the final FRCA syllabus so it is important to know the management of posterior fossa cases.

Jagannathan, S. and Krovvidi, H. (2014) Anaesthetic considerations for posterior fossa surgery. *CEACCP*, **14(5):** 202–206.

CRQ 3: answer guidance

Syllabus	OB_IS_02, OB_IK_01
Question type	Easy: pass mark 14
Topic	**Hypertensive disorders in pregnancy**
Aim	To recall the diagnosis and initial treatment of the hypertensive disorders of pregnancy.
Pass requirements	Correctly recall the first-line treatment for severe pre-eclampsia/eclampsia.

Q	Answer	Marks	Guidance
a	• >140mmHg systolic, >90mmHg diastolic or both together • confirmed on two separate occasions at least 4 hours apart	1 1	This is according to the American College of Obstetricians and Gynecologists.
b	Chronic hypertension becomes gestational hypertension when its onset is after 20 weeks' gestation	1	Once the patient is past the point of 20 weeks it becomes gestational in nature.
c	New onset hypertension (SBP >140mmHg, DBP >90mmHg) after 20 weeks, accompanied by one or more of the following features: • proteinuria • other maternal organ dysfunction (AKI, liver involvement, neurological complications, haematological complications) • uteroplacental dysfunction (restricted growth, absent Doppler)	1 2	1 mark for new onset hypertension after 20 weeks, then 1 mark each for either proteinuria/organ dysfunction/uteroplacental dysfunction. This may also include changes in liver function tests or change in haematological blood tests. HELLP syndrome is also included here.
d	• Prior pre-eclampsia • Chronic hypertension • Maternal BMI >30 • Pregestational diabetes mellitus • Antiphospholipid syndrome/lupus • Assisted reproduction • Primiparity • Interpregnancy interval >5 years or change of paternity • Advanced maternal age >40 • Family history of pre-eclampsia • Multiple gestation • CKD	5	1 mark per correct answer. The top six factors are stronger risk factors, whereas the bottom six are moderate risk factors.

Q	Answer	Marks	Guidance
e	• Labetalol 100mg BD (200mg/day) • Nifedipine 10mg OD • Methyldopa 250mcg BD	2	Must include dose to get the mark. 1 mark per correct answer. Labetalol can be up-titrated up to 800mg per day Nifedipine can be up-titrated to max 90mg OD Methyldopa can be titrated up to 3mg daily Patients should be started on the lowest dose and titrated up to effect.
f	• Severe headache • Signs of cerebral irritability • Clonus • Visual disturbance	3	1 mark per correct answer. Can also accept vomiting or other localising neurological signs that might suggest ICB.
g	• Magnesium sulfate • Initial loading dose 4–6g IV over 20–30 mins • Continuous infusion of 1–2g/hr	1 1 1	This should continue until 24 hours post delivery.
h	The most recent bloods should be within the last 6 hours.	1	Coagulopathy is one of the contraindications of neuraxial block and if the patient shows any coagulopathy, this should be undertaken with extreme caution.

Maternal hypertensive disorders is a key part of the primary FRCA curriculum. It should not be forgotten as part of the essential knowledge needed for the final, as it is likely you will encounter patients with hypertensive disorders throughout your career. The key step in management is getting the blood pressure under control to prevent intracerebral haemorrhages and stroke. A useful tool in patients who present for delivery is epidural anaesthesia, as this will prevent hypertensive surges associated with pain and sympathetic stimulation. It is important to remember these patients can become coagulopathic and so it is important to have up-to-date blood tests before commencing.

Goddard, J., Wee, M. and Vinayakarao, L. (2020) Update on hypertensive disorders in pregnancy. BJA Education, 20(12): 411–416.

Leslie, D. and Collis, R. (2016) Hypertensive disorders in pregnancy. BJA Education, 16(1): 33–37.

CRQ 4: answer guidance

Syllabus	CT_IK_02, PR_IK_05
Question type	Hard: pass mark 10
Topic	**Cardioplegia**
Aim	To understand the components of cardioplegia solution and their physiological roles.
Pass requirements	List the complications associated with cardioplegia solution.

Q	Answer	Marks	Guidance
a	• Prompt arrest of electromechanical activity, which helps facilitate surgery • Myocardial protection and prevention of myocardial cell death • Buffers ischaemic acidosis • Combats intracellular ion losses	3	1 mark per correct answer. Each of these is important in considering the composition of the cardioplegia solution.
b	**Calcium:** maintains cell membrane integrity	2	NB: Maximum marks 8. Other possible additives include: adenosine, arginine, NAC, nicorandil, aspartate, glutamate.
	Magnesium: reduces risk of peri-operative arrhythmia and prevents calcium overload; stabilises myocardial membrane	2	
	Mannitol: reduces tissue oedema by raising osmolarity	2	
	Bicarbonate: to resist large changes in pH and prevent acidaemia	2	
	Procaine: decreases cell excitability	2	
c	• Better H^+ ion buffering • Oxygen-carrying capacity of blood • Free radical scavenging ability of blood • Reduced myocardial oedema • Improved microvascular flow • Delivery of other nutrients	3	1 mark per correct answer. Blood cardioplegia may not be of much use in oxygen delivery due to change of the oxygen dissociation curve. Nevertheless it is considered possibly more physiological.
d	• Complications due to access (bleeding/damage to adjacent structures) • Inadequate protection of the myocardium due to failures during administration • Ischaemic injury due to lack of oxygen delivery • Air embolism due to air within the cardioplegia solution • Fluid overload • Myocardial oedema	3	1 mark per correct answer. Can accept any other relevant complication; however, these are the most common.
e	**Anterograde:** coronary arteries/ coronary ostia	1	These are the most common placements.
	Retrograde: coronary sinus	1	
f	To rule out aortic regurgitation, which would mean that retrograde cardioplegia is unsafe.	1	TOE should be performed prior to any bypass, as not only does it help with cardioplegia placement, it may also detect other valvular or contractile abnormalities.

CRQs and SBAs for the Final FRCA

Cardioplegia is a fairly old technique for inducing cardiac arrest for cardiac bypass operations and its use can be associated with multiple complications (however, in most cases it is a safe technique). In reality, the cardioplegia solution is controlled primarily by the perfusionist in liaison with the operating surgeon, but it is important to be aware of any possible complications.

Machin, D. and Allsager, C. (2006) Principles of cardiopulmonary bypass. *CEACCP*, **6(5):** 176–181.

Scott, T. and Swanevelder, J. (2009) Perioperative myocardial protection. *CEACCP*, **9(3):** 97–101.

CRQ 5: answer guidance

Syllabus	PM_IK_04, PM_IK_07, PM_IK_08
Question type	Easy: pass mark 14
Topic	**Chronic back pain**
Aim	To be able to diagnose and assess patients who present with lower back pain.
Pass requirements	Recall the red flags in lower back pain that require further investigation or management.

Q	Answer	Marks	Guidance
a	• Pain between the lower costal margins and the gluteal folds • lasting more than 3 months	1 1	
b	• Unilateral leg pain radiating below the knee (which is more severe than the back pain) • Dermatomal numbness, paraesthesia and/or muscle weakness • Positive straight leg raise test • Extensor plantar response	2	1 mark per correct answer.
c	• Signs of nerve root involvement • Ongoing compensation claim • Long absence from work • Psychological distress or depression • Smoking • Poor physical fitness • Obesity	4	1 mark per correct answer.

Q	Answer	Marks	Guidance
d	• Age <20 at presentation • Age >55 at presentation • History of significant trauma • Constant progressive thoracic pain • Past history of significant medical comorbidity (cancer, steroid therapy, IV drug abuse, HIV infection) • Unexplained weight loss • Systemically unwell • Cauda equina syndrome • Structural deformity (e.g. step deformity) • Marked restriction of lumbar flexion (<5cm total flexion) • Non-mechanical pain • Point tenderness over a vertebral body • Sudden onset, severe pain relieved by lying down	6	1 mark per correct answer. These can be reviewed in the NICE guidelines. Any reasonable answer from the guidelines can be accepted.
e	• Ibuprofen 400mg TDS • Omeprazole 20mg OD	1 1	NICE recommends an NSAID plus gastro-protection as first-line treatment. Codeine +/– paracetamol should be offered if NSAIDs are contraindicated or not tolerated.
f	• Advise that the cause of their pain is not serious • Give advice on simple exercises • Local heat therapy (e.g. heat pads) • Resume/maintain normal activities • Advise on adaptations to allow return to work	4	1 mark per correct answer. Accept 'avoid bed rest'.

Back pain is a common cause of referral to chronic pain clinics, but you may meet patients with back pain in other settings. This question is testing your ability to provide advice to an admitting team – ruling out concerning diagnoses (which the admitting team may have missed) and provide an initial management plan.

Jackson, M. and Simpson, K. (2006) Chronic back pain. *CEACCP*, **6(4):** 152–155.

NICE (2020) *Back pain – low (without radiculopathy)*. Available at: https://cks.nice.org.uk/topics/back-pain-low-without-radiculopathy/ (accessed 10 Feb 2022).

CRQ 6: answer guidance

Syllabus	PA_IK_01, PA_IK_11, PA_IK_12, PA_IK_14
Question type	Easy: pass mark 14
Topic	**Pyloric stenosis**
Aim	To be able to recall the presentation and salient management factors of pyloric stenosis in neonates.
Pass requirements	Candidates should show an appreciation of the challenges of anaesthesia of the infant and, in particular, in the context of the physiological derangement of pyloric stenosis. They should be able to give an initial treatment strategy and show knowledge of strategies to prevent the major complications of this surgery.

Q	Answer	Marks	Guidance
a	10%	1	Can accept between 7.5% and 12.5%.
b	Expedited	1	Can accept 'within days'. Can also accept a code 3 as per the NCEPOD codes of urgency.
c	**Resuscitation:** • Hartmann's solution or 0.9% NaCl • 20ml/kg **Maintenance:** • 0.45% NaCl with 5% dextrose and 20mmol/L KCl • 150ml/day	1 1 1	1 mark for both fluid and volume (no half marks). Can accept any isotonic fluid or total volumes calculated for age.
d	• Loss into vomited gastric secretions • Exchange for hydrogen ions in the kidney	1 1	This is an attempt to compensate for the alkalosis.
e	• Pre-operative insertion of NG tube • 4-quadrant aspiration of NG tube • Ultrasound assessment of gastric contents • Avoidance of hypoxaemia • Neuromuscular blockade	3	1 mark per correct answer.
f	• Shorter length of stay • Less post-operative pain • Shorter time to full feeds	2	1 mark per correct answer.
g	• Paracetamol 15mg/kg 6-hourly • Local anaesthetic infiltration OR • Rectus sheath block OR • Transversus abdominus plane (TAP) block	2	1 mark per correct answer.

Q	Answer	Marks	Guidance
h	• Pre-term delivery • Age <4 weeks • Anaemia • Use of general anaesthesia • Use of opiate analgesia • Low birth weight • History of apnoeic episodes • Oxygen therapy • Metabolic derangements • Cardiac, metabolic or hepatic comorbidities	6	1 mark per correct answer.

The biochemical abnormalities associated with and anaesthetic management of pyloric stenosis are common topics of questioning in both the written and SOE portions of the FRCA final examination. This case is so often used because it combines two challenging aspects of management: neonatal anaesthesia and the physiology of the biochemical derangements. You should be able to explain with confidence the causes of the classical hypochloraemic hypokalaemic metabolic alkalosis and why paradoxical aciduria can be present. Think about the likely anaesthetic risks of any patient with gastric outlet obstruction or any neonate, and how you might reduce them.

Craig, R. and Deely, A. (2018) Anaesthesia for pyloromyotomy. *BJA Education*, **18(6):** 173–177.

CRQ 7: answer guidance

Syllabus	PB_IK_02, CT_IK_03, OB_IS_11
Question type	Hard: pass mark 10
Topic	**Cardiomyopathy in pregnancy**
Aim	To understand the management of complex cardiac patients who present for anaesthesia in pregnancy.
Pass requirements	Describe the key anaesthetic goals in the management of the patient with cardiomyopathy.

Q	Answer	Marks	Guidance
a	• A myocardial disorder where the heart muscle is structurally and functionally abnormal • in the absence of coronary artery disease, hypertension, valvular heart disease and congenital heart disease sufficient to cause the observed abnormality	1 1	All cardiac diseases do not have to be listed but could be summarised into a point. There have been multiple definitions of cardiomyopathy but this is the most recent, as per the 2007 European Society of Cardiology.

Q	Answer	Marks	Guidance
b	**Dilated cardiomyopathy:** *Aetiology*: idiopathic (⅔rds), familial association, post-viral, cardiotoxic agents (e.g. chemo) and due to underlying disease *Pathophysiology*: increasing <u>systolic dysfunction</u> with progressive enlargement of one or both ventricles, leading to <u>overall reduction in stroke volume</u> *Clinical features*: signs of heart failure, dyspnoea, fatigue, ascites, peripheral oedema, arrhythmia, death	3	Overall a candidate should be able to have a good understanding of all three features of each type of cardiomyopathy. For certain types there are multiple signs and symptoms, so an examiner should expect 2–3 features to give the mark. Underlined features are essential to gain the mark.
	Hypertrophic cardiomyopathy: *Aetiology*: <u>inherited (autosomal dominant)</u> *Pathophysiology*: hypertrophy in heart muscle causes <u>diastolic impairment</u>. Extracellular fibrosis causes ventricular impairment and further diastolic impairment. Systolic function remains normal until late in disease *Clinical features*: usually asymptomatic, angina pectoris, syncope, sudden cardiac death	3	
	Restrictive cardiomyopathy: *Aetiology*: primary (idiopathic), secondary (amyloid, sarcoid, haemochromatosis, IHD, hypertension, valvular disease) *Pathophysiology*: fibrotic/infiltrative changes to the myocardium and subendocardium which <u>reduce compliance</u> and elevate end diastolic pressure *Clinical features*: dyspnoea, orthopnoea, fatigue, palpitations, oedema, chest pain (symptoms of biventricular failure). May have audible third heart sound, raised JVP, systolic murmur	3	

Q	Answer	Marks	Guidance
c	• Angiotensin-converting enzyme inhibitors • Angiotensin II receptor blockers • Beta blockers • Aldosterone inhibitors • Atrial natriuretic peptides • Anticoagulants	2	1 mark per pair. ACE inhibitors reduce disease progression but these would usually be stopped prior to attempted conception, due to risks to the foetus. Beta blockers and aldosterone inhibitors reduce mortality in heart failure. No half marks.
d	• Avoid myocardial depression • Maintain adequate preload and prevent increases in afterload • Avoid tachycardia or arrhythmias and treat promptly • Prevent sudden hypotension	1 1 1 1	Much of this can be achieved by careful titration of anaesthetic agents. Use of regional techniques can be useful here as there may be minimal haemodynamic changes. Central block may also reduce afterload.
e	• The patient should be offered an early epidural • This will prevent large changes in afterload during the contraction stage due to circulating adrenaline • It will facilitate conversion to caesarean section via epidural top-up, preventing large haemodynamic changes	1 1 1	This will go in keeping with maintaining the key anaesthetic goals, as per the previous question. In practice care must be taken that the patient is not on anticoagulants, as this may prevent neuraxial anaesthesia. It is also not unreasonable that the patient may be offered an ICD prior to labour.

Cardiomyopathy in pregnancy can be challenging to manage and requires a great deal of multidisciplinary input prior to the patient presenting in labour. Often there is liaison between obstetricians, cardiologists, anaesthetists and the patient to facilitate as smooth a delivery as possible. Ideally these patients will be managed in a tertiary centre and should have invasive monitoring in the peri-partum phase. The anaesthetic goals for managing a patient in labour should be the same as those for any other operation, but there are certain subtle changes. The ability to place neuraxial anaesthesia early can be beneficial here, as it can help not only in the labour phase but also if there is a conversion to operative management; this should therefore always be discussed with anyone presenting with severe cardiac disease. It may even be prudent to manage the patient in cardiac theatres with the assistance of a skilled cardiac anaesthetist if the disease is severe.

Burt, C. and Durbridge, J. (2009) Management of cardiac disease in pregnancy. *CEACCP*, **9(2):** 44–47.

Ibrahim, I. and Sharma, V. (2017) Cardiomyopathy and anaesthesia. *BJA Education*, **17(11):** 363–369.

CRQs and SBAs for the Final FRCA

CRQ 8: answer guidance

Syllabus	AM_IK_03, MK_IT_02
Question type	Medium: pass mark 12
Topic	**Management of blunt and penetrating neck trauma**
Aim	To be able to form an appropriate airway management plan for patients with neck trauma, both penetrating and blunt.
Pass requirements	Identify the contents of the carotid sheath.

Q	Answer	Marks	Guidance
a	• Common carotid artery • Internal jugular vein • Vagus nerve • Recurrent laryngeal nerve • Deep cervical lymph nodes • Ansa cervicalis	4	1 mark per correct answer. Must state common carotid artery (although parts of the internal carotid artery and external are contained, they are not main structures). The ansa cervicalis is embedded in the anterior wall.
b	• Airway compromise • Massive subcutaneous emphysema • Bubbling or sucking neck wounds • Large volume haematemesis • Large volume haemoptysis	4	1 mark per correct answer. These are hard signs, although there may be soft signs.
c	• Direct placement of tracheal tube through the deficit using a fibrescope • Awake fibre-optic intubation • Awake surgical tracheostomy under local anaesthesia • Modified RSI using direct or videolaryngoscopy	3	1 mark per correct answer. Awake fibre-optic intubation is still a choice in trauma as long as the patient is cooperative and stable enough to perform it. All options should be done in theatre with an experienced ENT/Max Fax surgeon present.
d	• Can dislodge fractured cartilage (cricoid, thyroid, cricoid) • Can exit through defect, creating a false passage • Could worsen bleeding	2	1 mark per correct answer Can also include mark for 'positive pressure in false passage can distort anatomy further'.
e	Tube should be placed with the cuff below the defect	1	Cuff should be mentioned to gain mark.

Q	Answer	Marks	Guidance
f	• Conventional front of neck access, as this can worsen already distorted anatomy and make surgical access difficult • Positive pressure ventilation through supraglottic or facemask, as this may lead to worsening surgical emphysema • Cricoid pressure, as it may not compress the oesophagus completely and can worsen bleeding	3	1 mark per correct answer These should all be avoided; however, in very specific circumstances (i.e. arrest/periarrest) it may be appropriate to perform facemask ventilation or FONA.
g	• Respiratory distress • Ecchymosis of the neck • Surgical emphysema around the neck • Tracheal deviation • Haemoptysis • Rapidly extending haematoma	3	1 mark per correct answer. Stridor may also be a possible answer, although not strictly an examination finding.

Neck trauma is not a common presentation to A&E but could still present anywhere in the country, not just major trauma centres. It is thus essential to have a good knowledge of this type of presentation and management. Many of these answers come with caveats – an ENT surgeon is readily available; however, this may not always be the case. This is especially relevant regarding when you would or would not perform FONA or face-mask ventilation. In reality it is a judgement call at the time with senior and experienced assistance.

Shilston, J., Evans D.L., Simons, A. and Evans, D.A. (2021) Initial management of blunt and penetrating neck trauma. *BJA Education*, **21(9):** 329–335.

CRQ 9: answer guidance

Syllabus	PL_IK_03, PL_IK_03
Question type	Hard: pass mark 10
Topic	**Anaesthesia for breast surgery and flap reconstruction**
Aim	To understand the physiological factors that govern blood flow and anaesthesia for successful flap surgery.
Pass requirements	Explain how a free flap is monitored post-operatively in HDU.

Q	Answer	Marks	Guidance
a	**Pedicled:** • Latissimus dorsi	1	These are the most common types of autologous flap.
	Non-pedicled (free flap): • Transverse rectus abdominis myocutaneous (TRAM) • Deep inferior epigastric perforator (DIEP)	1 1	Using the DIEP method spares the rectus muscle and therefore preserves abdominal strength.

Q	Answer	Marks	Guidance
b	• Raising of the flap via dissection to separate out blood vessels • Microvascular anastomosis • Insetting of flap and shaping of tissue	1 1 1	These are the stages in a free flap. Pedicled flapping follows a slightly different pattern due to the pedicle remaining *in situ*. Does not necessarily need to be in correct order to gain mark. Vascular anastomosis would be acceptable.
c	• Anaerobic metabolism leading to a rise in lactate • A decrease in intracellular pH • Increase in calcium levels • Increase in pro-inflammatory mediator levels	3	1 mark per correct answer. This all occurs during the primary ischaemia phase and the damage caused is proportional to the duration of ischaemia.
d	0.2ml/min per 100g tissue	1	This is five times less than muscle, so TRAM flaps are more sensitive to ischaemia than DIEP.
e	• Nicotine-induced vasoconstriction • Carbon monoxide-related tissue hypoxia • Increased blood coagulability	1 1 1	Can also accept 'increased platelet aggregation' as this causes increased coagulability.
f	• Maintain systemic arterial pressure to ensure flap perfusion • Patient temperature control • Normovolaemia • Maintain normal Hb level	3	1 mark per correct answer. This is based on the Hagen–Poiseuille equation, which can be manipulated to ensure adequate perfusion. Overzealous fluid use will cause tissue oedema and ultimately flap failure.
g	Flap colour Capillary refill time Skin turgor Skin temperature Bleeding on pinprick	4	1 mark per correct answer. Can also accept 'Doppler measurement' as this is often used to assess perforator blood vessels.

Although primarily the survival of a flap is based on good surgical technique, there are many anaesthetic factors that can help in ensuring flap survival. The Hagen–Poiseuille equation can be manipulated to give the best blood flow and therefore oxygen delivery to the free flap. Length of vessel is fixed but everything else can be manipulated to ensure best survival. Overzealous transfusion of blood or fluid should be avoided in these cases to prevent oedema; however, insidious haemorrhage is possible, and regular Hb checks may be necessary.

Nimalan, N., Branford, O. and Stocks, G. (2016) Anaesthesia for free flap breast reconstruction. *BJA Education*, **16(5):** 162–166.

Sherwin, A. and Buggy, D. (2018) Anaesthesia for breast surgery. *BJA Education*, **18(11):** 342–348.

CRQ 10: answer guidance

Syllabus	PR_IK_03
Question type	Easy: pass mark 14
Topic	**Critical incidents (MH)**
Aim	To understand the pathophysiology of malignant hyperthermia.
Pass requirements	Confidently describe the clinical management of MH.

Q	Answer	Marks	Guidance
a	• Mechanical: inadequate fresh gas flow, insufficient ventilation, inappropriate breathing circuit, machine malfunction • Anaesthetic: inadequate anaesthesia and/or analgesia, anaphylaxis, cerebral ischaemia • Patient-related: malignant hyperthermia, phaeochromocytoma, neuromuscular disorders, pre-existing infection, sepsis • Idiosyncratic: anaphylaxis	4	1 mark per correct answer. MH has a wide differential and this list is not exhaustive.
b	*Susceptibility*: abnormality most commonly in the ryanodine receptor on the sarcoplasmic reticulum	2	1 mark for each trigger to maximum 4.
	Trigger: most commonly succinylcholine or volatiles induce calcium release Calcium triggers dysregulated muscle fibre contraction CO_2 release Glycogen breakdown and lactate release Potassium released from intracellular stores	4	

Q	Answer	Marks	Guidance
c	*Anaesthetic*: stop volatiles, remove vaporiser, hyperventilate with 100% oxygen; charcoal filters, clean anaesthetic machine *Dantrolene* (starting dose 2.5mg/kg) *Hyperthermia*: discontinue warming and start active cooling *Monitoring*: continue CO_2 monitorings, cardiac monitoring *Hyperkalaemia*: treat with IV insulin/dextrose *Acidosis*: hyperventilate +/– HCO_3 if pH <7.2 *Arrhythmias*: monitor, treat tachycardia with beta blocker *AKI*: fluids +/– filtration *DIC*: monitoring and reversal of coagulopathy *Ongoing care*: usually requires ICU admission	8	1 mark per correct answer. To gain mark for dantrolene, at least 1 dose should be mentioned.
d	• Genetic testing • Muscle biopsy	1 1	Can accept caffeine/halothane testing.

Despite clinically being very rare, MH is a condition most anaesthetists are expected to have a sound knowledge of. This is mainly because it doesn't really present in many other situations or scenarios. Most anaesthetic machines will have a MH flowchart to follow if the situation ever does arise, and team management is important (it is likely at least two people will have to spend time mixing the dantrolene). Treated, it has a high likelihood of a good outcome; without treatment, mortality is high.

Gupta, P. and Hopkins, P. (2017) Diagnosis and management of malignant hyperthermia. *BJA Education*, **17(17):** 249–254.

CRQ 11: answer guidance

Syllabus	OP_IK_01, OP_IK_04, OP_IK_06
Question type	Moderate: pass mark 12
Topic	**Regional anaesthesia for ophthalmic surgery**
Aim	To understand the indications for, performance of, and risks involved in ophthalmic regional anaesthesia.
Pass requirements	Recall the relevant anatomy for ophthalmic anaesthesia.

Q	Answer	Marks	Guidance
a	1: cornea 2: Tenon's capsule 3: fovea 4: optic nerve 5: vitreous humour 6: sclera	3	1 mark per pair. No half marks.
b	• Sub-Tenon's: blunt • Peribulbar: sharp • Retrobulbar: sharp	3	1 mark per correct answer. Must be able to correctly identify sharp or blunt for full marks.
c	*Pressure*: 10–20mmHg *Factors*: • Change in intraocular contents • Scleral rigidity • External pressure on the globe	1 3	1 mark for each factor.
d	i. Yes. ii. As per guidelines, no starvation required for sedation with the aim of anxiolysis	1 1	Starvation is not clinically indicated for sedation for anxiolysis, where verbal contact with the patient should be able to be maintained.
e	*Cause*: parasympathetically mediated – traction on globe or pressure on globe *Afferent pathway*: signals pass via trigeminal nerve to medulla *Efferent pathway*: efferent fibres pass via vagus nerve to SA node	2 2 2	2 marks per correct pathway.
f	• Patient refusal • Allergy to local anaesthetic • Localised sepsis • Grossly abnormal coagulation • Inability to lie still (e.g. tremor, confusion) • Difficulties communicating • Poor compliance with instructions • Perforated globe or trauma	2	1 mark per pair of correct answers.

Ophthalmic anaesthesia is something that many candidates will not have a great deal of experience in; however, it is important to know the basics. An understanding of anatomy and intra-ocular pressure is an essential footing for all ophthalmic anaesthesia. A good way of remembering factors that influence IOP is that they are very similar to those governing ICP.

Anker, R. and Kaur, N. (2017) Regional anaesthesia for ophthalmic surgery. *BJA Education*, **17(7):** 221–227.

CRQ 12: answer guidance

Syllabus	EN_IK_03, EN_IK_13, EN_IK_16
Question type	Hard: pass mark 10
Topic	**Head and neck cancer surgery**
Aim	To understand the anaesthetic implications for head and neck surgery in cancer patients.
Pass requirements	Have a general understanding for the procedures involved in head and neck surgery.

Q	Answer	Marks	Guidance
a	• Smoking • Alcohol excess • Chewing tobacco • Poor oral hygiene • Exposure to wood dust • HPV infection	3	1 mark per correct answer. Can accept 'occupational exposure'.
b	**Patient:** • Higher incidence of alcohol abuse; may need admission for detox or management of withdrawal • Risk of refeeding syndrome should be anticipated and pre-empted • Difficult airway anticipated (radiotherapy, obstruction) **Environmental:** • Patient supine with 15–20 degrees head up to improve venous drainage • Long ventilator tubing/IV lines • Shared airway with possible obstruction – review of imaging or as a minimum FNE prior to intubation if lesion at level of cords essential • Temperature management: essential when only a small area is exposed for prolonged procedures. Peripheral measurement avoids damaging tumour or obstructing surgical field. Free flaps: no more than 1.5°C difference between bladder temp and flap temp **Anaesthetic:** • Provision of controlled blood pressure, most commonly with use of remifentanil: blunting of haemodynamic response to stimulating surgery	5	1 mark per correct answer. There can be some general overlap between patient/environmental/anaesthetic so can accept in any category.

Q	Answer	Marks	Guidance
c	**MLT and IPPV** *Advantages*: • Airway secure with cuffed tube • Specialist equipment and experience not required • Clear visualisation of ant. ⅔ of larynx *Disadvantages*: • Obstructed view of post. ⅓ of larynx • Risk of fire with use of laser • High resistance tube due to diameter **Supraglottic jet** *Advantages*: Optimal surgical access *Disadvantages*: • Entrained air leads to gastric distension • Can become misaligned easily • No CO_2 monitoring • No airway protection • Vocal cords move with ventilation • Potential for tumour seeding • Barotrauma risk • Unable to deliver volatiles **Subglottic jet** *Advantages*: • Minimal movement of vocal cords • Efficiency increased compared to supraglottic *Disadvantages*: • Unable to deliver volatiles • Greater risk of barotrauma • Unsecure airway • No CO_2 monitoring	6	1 mark per correct answer. For full marks should not mention same disadvantage in both types of jet ventilation.
d	• Tracheostomy • Remain intubated if using MLT	1 1	Can also accept 'leak test'.
e	• Pain (moderate, managed with simple analgesia and IV or s/c routes if unable to swallow) • Tracheostomy (coughing and irritation – can use nebulised 4% lidocaine) • Specialist nursing • Anticoagulation and haematocrit reduced to 30–35% • Respiratory distress/coughing	4	1 mark per correct answer.

This is a challenging topic, as jet ventilation is a higher level skill. However, candidates would be expected to know the reasons for using it rather than another form of airway management and the disadvantages associated with it.

Ahmed-Nusrath, A. (2017) Anaesthesia for head and neck cancer surgery. *BJA Education*, **17(12):** 383–389.

SBA 1: answer = D – Stop ventilation

Airway and non-airway fires are a risk of laser surgery. In the event of a laser-induced airway fire, the sequence of events should be as follows:
1. Discontinue laser surgery and make surgeon aware
2. Stop ventilation
3. Disconnect the O_2 source
4. Remove burnt ETT
5. Douse operating site with water
6. Reinstate ventilation once fire arrested
7. Perform bronchoscopy thereafter.

Simpson, E. (2012) The basic principles of laser technology, uses and safety measures in anaesthesia. *Anaesthesia Tutorial of the Week,* **255**.

SBA 2: answer = B – Sickle cell disease

Sickle cell disease is the only complete contraindication, along with untreated/uncontrolled polycythaemia rubra vera. This is because these conditions prevent graft survival by causing microvascular sludging. All of the others could be relative contraindications.

Ahmed-Nusrath, A. (2017) Anaesthesia for head and neck cancer surgery. *BJA Education,* **17(12):** 383–389.

SBA 3: answer = B – Microvascular decompression

Patients who have trigeminal neuralgia resistant to pharmacological therapy should be considered for invasive procedures. Microvascular decompression is associated with a relapse rate of around 30–40% at 10 years but has the best long-term pain relief of the procedures described. This remains a major neurosurgical procedure with associated complications, which should be taken into consideration. Peripheral techniques (neurectomy and neurolysis) often last up to 1 year, and at the level of the Gasserian ganglion (chemical ablation) benefit lasts 4–5 years in 50% of patients. Terminal nerve branch blockade is unlikely to be of any benefit.

Vasappa, C., Kapur, S. and Krovvidi, H. (2016) Trigeminal neuralgia. *BJA Education,* **16(10):** 353–356.

SBA 4: answer = D – 8

The APGAR score is formed of 5 distinct categories, each scored between 0 and 2.

Appearance: a blue baby is 0, blue extremities are 1, and pink is 2.
Pulse: >100bpm is 2, <100 is 1 and absent is 0.
Grimace: when stimulated, if the baby responds promptly this is 2, minimal response is 1, and no response is 0.
Activity: active motion is 2, some flexion is 1, and flaccidity is 0.
Respiratory: no respiration is 0, irregular/weak respiration is 1, and a vigorous cry is 2.

The baby described has an APGAR score of 8, which means that the baby was born in good condition.

Finster, M., Wood, M. and Raja, S. (2005) The APGAR score has survived the test of time. *Anaesthesiology,* **102:** 855–857.

SBA 5: answer = E – Isotope perfusion scanning

If initial investigations suggest significant pulmonary hypertension, it is important to exclude thromboembolism as a cause. This is because it can be rapidly treated if diagnosed. Isotope perfusion scanning is the most sensitive way of excluding pulmonary emboli as a cause; however, in practice it may not be convenient to obtain. As an alternative a CTPA can be used. Right-heart catheterisation will give accurate pressures but will not exclude pulmonary emboli. TTE or TOE may show presence of a clot but are user-dependent.

Condcliffe, R. and Kiely, D. (2017) Critical care management of pulmonary hypertension. *BJA Education*, **17(7):** 228–234.

SBA 6: answer = B – No intervention required

The patient has a 2nd-degree AV block (Mobitz Type I block). This usually appears after the patient has suffered an MI, but is usually self-limiting. If the patient is asymptomatic and otherwise well there is no need for further investigation or intervention. If the patient is symptomatic, they will need referral to a cardiologist or permanent pacemaker insertion due to the risk of developing 2:1 block and haemodynamic instability.

Dua, N. and Kumra, V. (2007) Management of perioperative arrhythmias. *Indian Journal of Anaesthesia*, **51(4):** 310–323.

SBA 7: answer = A – 1.5ml/kg of 20% lipid emulsion (Intralipid) bolus followed by an infusion of 15ml/kg/hour

This patient has symptoms suggestive of local anaesthetic toxicity and will need to be treated immediately with intravenous lipid emulsion. There is nothing to suggest that the patient has airway or ventilatory compromise, so at this time intubation would not be the best option. Propofol should not be used as a lipid sink. The patient does not have signs of eclampsia so magnesium is not indicated, nor is there any suggestion that the patient has lost output and requires CPR. The left lateral position would be ineffective as treatment for the root cause here.

Christie, L., Picard, J. and Weinberg, G. (2015) Local anaesthetic systemic toxicity. *BJA Education*, **15(3):** 136–142.

SBA 8: answer = C – CSE with low dose spinal

The patient has presented unexpectedly in labour, but has also had one foetal bradycardia – making the caesarean section more urgent. With aortic stenosis, it is safer to avoid any method of anaesthesia that will result in haemodynamic instability or hypotension, as the patient has a fixed cardiac output. This means that IV induction, as well as a single-shot spinal anaesthetic, would be relatively contraindicated. Due to the more urgent nature of the surgery it would be more prudent to perform a CSE rather than an epidural alone, as this may take some time to develop the required block. These patients should have an arterial line inserted for beat-to-beat blood pressure monitoring to facilitate early intervention.

Burt, C. and Durbridge, J. (2009) Management of cardiac disease in pregnancy. *CEACCP*, **9(2):** 44–47.

SBA 9: answer = E – Transthoracic Doppler

Transoesophageal echocardiography and Doppler are the most sensitive for recognising venous air embolism. However, they are not often used due to increased complications associated with the insertion of the TOE probe and the skill required to obtain and interpret images. Precordial Doppler is the next best alternative and can detect as little as 0.015ml/kg/min of intra-cardiac air. A loss of etCO$_2$ can be an indicator of VAE but may not be sensitive, and the same can be said for a drop in mean arterial pressure. NIRS and jugular bulb saturations can be a marker of cerebral perfusion, but they are not necessarily sensitive for the detection of VAE.

Jagannathan, S. and Krovvidi, H. (2014) Anaesthetic considerations for posterior fossa surgery. *CEACCP*, **14(5):** 202–206.

SBA 10: answer = A – Atropine

After transplantation, the heart's response to circulating catecholamines is attenuated and delayed. There is loss of direct sympathetic input from the sympathetic ganglion and loss of parasympathetic input from the vagus nerve. As a result, atropine will have no effect on heart rate. Other indirectly acting sympathomimetics such as ephedrine should be avoided due to unpredictable effects.

Edwards, S., Allen, S. and Sidebotham, D. (2021) Anaesthesia for heart transplantation. *BJA Education*, **21(8):** 284–291.

SBA 11: answer = A – Must only be initiated by the anaesthetist performing the block

The 'SB4UB' process can be initiated by anyone (anaesthetist, ODP or other theatre staff). The rest are all essential parts of the process.

Safe Anaesthesia Liaison Group (SALG) and Regional Anaesthesia UK (RAUK) (2011) *Stop before you block*. Available at: www.ra-uk.org/index.php/stop-before-you-block (accessed 16 February 2022).

SBA 12: answer = D – Transverse spinous ligament

The integrity and stability of the spine are dependent on the combined function of a number of ligaments: the anterior longitudinal ligament for the anterior half of the intervertebral discs, the posterior longitudinal ligament for the posterior half of the intervertebral discs, and the posterior complex, which articulates with the spinous and transverse processes. The posterior complex consists of the interspinous ligament, the ligamentum flavum and the supraspinous ligament.

Bonner, S. and Smith, C. (2013) Initial management of acute spinal cord injury. *CEACCP*, **13(6):** 224–231.

SBA 13: answer = B – Resuscitative hysterotomy

If there is no return of spontaneous circulation by 4 minutes, a resuscitative hysterotomy (perimortem caesarean section) should be performed by 5 minutes – at the site of arrest if necessary. Atropine and amiodarone have no role in PEA as per ALS guidelines, and PEA is a non-shockable rhythm. Magnesium, uterotonics and neuraxial local anaesthetics must be stopped rather than commenced.

Madden, A. and Meng, M. (2020) Cardiopulmonary resuscitation in the pregnant patient. *BJA Education*, **20(8):** 252–258.

SBA 14: answer = E – Increased theta wave power

Adequate sevoflurane anaesthesia results in an increase in alpha, theta and slow delta wave power. An increase in beta wave power is associated with an inadequate plane of sevoflurane anaesthesia. Conversely, ketamine anaesthesia causes an increase in beta wave power, which is one reason why processed-EEG monitors do not reflect the depth of ketamine anaesthesia well. Burst suppression is likely to be associated with a deeper level of anaesthesia than 1.0 MAC in an otherwise fit, healthy person. The mention of propofol in this question can be largely disregarded, as the EEG manifestations of propofol anaesthesia are broadly similar to sevoflurane and in any case would have worn off after 1 hour.

Hajat, Z., Ahmad, N. and Andrzejowski, J. (2017) The role and limitations of EEG-based depth of anaesthesia monitoring in theatres and intensive care. *Anaesthesia*, **72(S1):** 38–47.

Kim, P., Fricchione, G., Brown, E. and Akeju, O. (2020) Role of electroencephalogram oscillations and the spectrogram in monitoring anaesthesia. *BJA Education*, **20(5):** 166–172.

SBA 15: answer = A – 10ml O_2/kg/min

All patients being considered for high-risk thoracic surgery should undergo CPEX testing as part of the pre-assessment work-up. The most valuable measurement in CPEX in this case is the peak oxygen consumption. A value >20 is considered fit for surgery, and >15 is considered to be in good physical fitness. A value below 10 is considered a contraindication for surgery.

Hackett, S., Jones, R. and Kapila, R. (2019) Anaesthesia for pneumonectomy. *BJA Education*, **19(9):** 297–304.

SBA 16: answer = B – Dexmedetomidine

All the options, except diclofenac, are accepted as potential additives to local anaesthetic mixtures to extend block duration. Adrenaline is commonly used, but is relatively contraindicated in patients with existing peripheral neuropathy – as would be in this case. Dexamethasone is likely to result in higher blood sugars, affecting wound healing, and there is some evidence of neurotoxicity *in vivo*. Magnesium is inconsistent, and has also been shown to have neurotoxic potential. Dexmedetomidine is a safer alternative, but caution with dosing is necessary to minimise sedation, hypotension and bradycardia.

Desai, N., Albrecht, E. and El-Boghdadly, K. (2019) Perineural adjuncts for peripheral nerve block. *BJA Education*, **19(9):** 276–282.

SBA 17: answer = B – T10

The vagal trunks descend through the diaphragm via the oesophageal hiatus, which occurs at the T10 level. Key structures that pass through the diaphragm include the inferior vena cava (T8) and descending aorta (T12).

King, W. and Dickinson, M. (2015) Oesophageal injury. *BJA Education*, **15(5):** 265–270.

SBA 18: answer = C – Adjusting the patient to 10 degrees Trendelenburg

Pharmacological techniques to optimise the operative field include increasing the depth of anaesthesia, labetalol, esmolol, remifentanil and magnesium – for which the recommended dose for the effect required is 50mg/kg IV over 5 minutes (see *Table 2* of below reference). Hypercarbia can induce vasodilation and increase arterial pressure. Minimising inspiratory time limits the raised intrathoracic pressure during positive pressure ventilation – which is responsible for restricting venous return. Minimising PEEP has the same effect. Trendelenburg (head down) position is not beneficial and promotes higher arterial pressures and venous pooling.

Pairaudeau, C. and Mendonca, C. (2019) Anaesthesia for major middle ear surgery. *BJA Education*, **19(5):** 136–143.

SBA 19: answer = D – Ramipril 1.25mg ON

Antihypertensives should continue in the peri-operative period, with the exception of angiotensin-converting enzyme inhibitors and angiotensin receptor blockers. Beta blockers are beneficial in patients with a history of myocardial infarction, but the stroke risk increases with high dosing. Clopidogrel and aspirin should both continue, and there is no significant increase in haematoma or haemorrhage when clopidogrel is taken with or without aspirin in the population.

Stoneham, M., Stamou, D. and Mason, J. (2015) Regional anaesthesia for carotid endarterectomy. *BJA*, **114(3):** 372–383.

SBA 20: answer = A – Amputation

Amputation has up to 85% incidence of chronic post-surgical pain (CPSP), which is the greatest of any surgical procedure. The exact aetiology of CPSP is not clear, as not all surgery associated with nerve damage is associated with CPSP. The optimal pain management of these patients is multimodal, with a combination of systemic and neuraxial techniques.

Searle, R. and Simpson, K. (2010) Chronic post-surgical pain. *CEACCP*, **10(1):** 12–14.

SBA 21: answer = C – 6–9%

These signs and symptoms are indicative of a child who is clinically dehydrated (has lost more than 5% of their weight in lost fluid) but not shocked. Shock is usually evident when the percentage dehydration is 10% or over. This child would be suitable for management with oral rehydration if tolerated. Remember that the normal ranges for observations are adjusted for age. In this case, he is mildly tachycardic and tachypnoeic but not hypotensive.

NICE (2009, updated 2018) *Diarrhoea and vomiting caused by gastroenteritis in under 5s: diagnosis and management* [CG 84]. Available at: https://www.nice.org.uk/guidance/cg84/resources/diarrhoea-and-vomiting-caused-by-gastroenteritis-in-under-5s-diagnosis-and-management-pdf-975688889029 (accessed 15 March 2022).

SBA 22: answer = A – Viral meningitis

The patient has viral meningitis, which can present with variable neurological symptoms. The CSF lymphocytosis should point to a viral cause, and although HIV encephalitis is possible, it is much less likely. The CSF glucose is greater than half the serum glucose, which is characteristic of viral meningitis.

Johnstone, C., Hall, A. and Hart, I. (2014) Common viral illnesses in intensive care: presentation, diagnosis and management. *CEACCP*, **14(5)**: 213–219.

SBA 23: answer = C – 5 days

Many patients who present for emergency neck of femur surgery are likely to have multiple comorbidities and will be on a variety of medications. The decision to perform a spinal anaesthetic or general anaesthetic will vary from case to case. If the patient has had fondaparinux together with ticagrelor, a spinal anaesthetic would not be appropriate acutely. However, if the patient has had ticagrelor only, it would be acceptable to perform a spinal anaesthetic 5 days after the last dose.

Association of Anaesthetists of Great Britain and Ireland; Obstetric Anaesthetists' Association; Regional Anaesthesia UK (2013) Regional anaesthesia and patients with abnormalities of coagulation. *Anaesthesia*, **68:** 966–972.

SBA 24: answer = D – Patients with malignant hyperthermia are at increased risk of serotonin syndrome

Although patients with malignant hyperthermia (MH) are not at increased risk of serotonin syndrome, it is still recommended that combinations of serotonergic drugs are avoided. This is because the symptoms of serotonin syndrome can easily be confused with those of MH. Anti-parkinsonian medication should be continued in all patients, as abrupt withdrawal can cause neuroleptic malignant syndrome. Whilst prophylactic dantrolene is not recommended, it should be readily available, as well as activated charcoal filters. These can be fitted to both limbs of the breathing circuit. TIVA can be used safely, providing the anaesthetist is confident with the use of TIVA and suxamethonium is not used.

Gupta, P., Bilmen, J. and Hopkins, P. (2021) Anaesthetic management of a known or suspected malignant hyperthermia susceptible patient. *BJA Education*, **21(6):** 218–224.

SBA 25: answer = C – The context-sensitive half-time is 5 minutes

The only incorrect statement is C. Although a common lockout time for remifentanil is 2 minutes, the CSHT is approximately 3 minutes, undergoing degradation by non-specific esterases.

Ronel, I. and Weiniger, C. (2019) Non-regional analgesia for labour: remifentanil in obstetrics. *BJA Education*, **19(11):** 357–361.

SBA 26: answer = A – Ventriculo-atrial shunt

Absolute contraindications to the sitting position include ventriculo-atrial shunt and right-to-left heart shunt. These conditions have a higher risk of devastating air embolism. The other options listed are relative contraindications, and should be considered on individual case merit and the ability to perform the surgery in an alternative position.

Jagannathan, S. and Krovvidi, H. (2014) Anaesthetic considerations for posterior fossa surgery. *CEACCP*, **14(5):** 202–206.

SBA 27: answer = E – No prophylaxis needed

There is no evidence for pre-operative prophylactic antibiotics for the prevention of infective endocarditis in the current NICE guidelines. In high-risk situations, such as operating in an infected cavity, discussion with the local microbiologist is indicated to determine the correct antimicrobial therapy.

NICE (2008) *Prophylaxis against infective endocarditis* [CG64]. Available at: www.nice.org.uk/guidance/cg64/evidence/full-guideline-pdf-196759981 (accessed 16 February 2022)

SBA 28: answer = C – 8 hours after tirofiban

Unfractionated heparin should be stopped preemptively 4 hours prior to central neuraxial blockade or with normal APTTR prior to blockade. Clopidogrel must be stopped 7 days prior, and ticagrelor stopped 5 days prior. Abciximab should be held for 48 hours.

Association of Anaesthetists of Great Britain and Ireland; Obstetric Anaesthetists' Association; Regional Anaesthesia UK (2013) Regional anaesthesia and patients with abnormalities of coagulation. *Anaesthesia*, **68:** 966–972.

SBA 29: answer = D – Superior laryngeal nerve

The cricothyroid muscle is the only tensor of the vocal cords and is supplied by the superior laryngeal nerve (branch of the vagus nerve). The recurrent laryngeal nerve innervates the intrinsic muscles of the larynx, but not the cricothyroid muscle. The intrinsic muscles are also supplied by the inferior laryngeal nerve, which provides sensory innervation to the larynx. The trigeminal nerve has no effect on the function of the larynx and there is no posterior laryngeal nerve.

Jones, O. and Barnes, S. (2020) *Laryngeal muscles*. TeachMe Anatomy [online]. Available at: https://teachmeanatomy.info/neck/viscera/larynx/muscles/ (accessed 18 February 2022).

SBA 30: answer = D – Unopposed action of the right cricothyroid muscle

Unilateral paramedian positioning of the vocal cords indicates injury to the ipsilateral recurrent laryngeal nerve (RLN). This could have been due to excessive cuff pressures/large tube size/use of bougie, etc. The end result is unopposed action of the right cricothyroid muscle (innervated by the external branch of the superior laryngeal nerve), as the RLN innervates the other intrinsic muscles of the larynx.

Evans, D., McGlashan, J. and Norris, A. (2015) Iatrogenic airway injury. *BJA Education*, **15(4):** 184–189.

SBA 31: answer = B – Cyanide poisoning

Cyanide poisoning is difficult to diagnose, as no rapid diagnostic tests are readily available. Suspicious history may include fires from plastics, vinyls and other synthetic materials, and a history of unconsciousness, hypoxia, haemodynamic instability (including cardiac arrest), convulsions, and fixed and unreactive pupils. To differentiate it from carbon monoxide poisoning, there would be a reduced arterio-venous O_2 gradient (<10%), raised anion gap acidosis and a lactate typically raised >7mmol/L.

Gill, P. and Martin, R. (2015) Smoke inhalation injury. *BJA Education*, **(15)3:** 143–148.

SBA 32: answer = B – Background: 3mg/hr. Bolus: 1.5mg

Converting oral morphine to IV requires division by a factor of 3 or 2 (based on oral to IV equipotency). This will provide a total IV daily dose, which is then divided by 24 (for each hour) to create a background infusion. A bolus requirement will be necessary, which should be 50% of the hourly bolus rate with a 5-minute lock out.

Simpson, G. and Jackson, M. (2017) Perioperative management of opioid-tolerant patients. *BJA Education*, **17(4):** 124–128.

SBA 33: answer = E – Laparoscopic surgery

Patients with a Fontan circulation lack the ability to increase preload, as the venous return is directed into the pulmonary circulation, rather than the heart. Thus they tolerate reductions in preload poorly. Preload is also dependent on maintaining a small pressure drop over the pulmonary circulation and so increases in pulmonary vascular resistance are poorly tolerated. Use of α-agonists, hypercarbia and alveolar hypoxia should be avoided as a result. All arrhythmias are poorly tolerated and should be aggressively managed with early defibrillation if necessary. Laparoscopic surgery is usually well tolerated, provided insufflation pressures are kept low (<10mmHg).

Nayak, S. and Booker, P. (2008) The Fontan circulation. *CEACCP*, **8(1):** 26–30.

SBA 34: answer = B – Restrictive lung disease

Indications for APRV include patients who are 'recruitable', patients with ARDS/multifocal pneumonia, patients likely to have further respiratory deterioration, patients who have failed a trial of proning, patients who have failed a trial of low-TV ventilation, obese patients and septic patients. Restrictive lung diseases are a relative contraindication for APRV.

Swindin, J., Sampson, C. and Howatson, A. (2020) Airway pressure release ventilation. *BJA Education*, **20(3):** 80–88.

SBA 35: answer = A – Transfusion-related acute lung injury (TRALI)

TRALI can occur up to 6 hours post-transfusion and typically presents as an acute respiratory distress syndrome (ARDS). Other causes of ARDS would need to be excluded prior to making a diagnosis, such as circulatory overload or myocardial disease. Due to the patient being febrile it is unlikely to be TACO. Non-haemolytic febrile reactions and non-ABO reactions would have been apparent earlier. Transfusion-associated graft-versus-host disease is very rare and so less likely with cross-matched blood.

Maxwell, M. and Wilson, M. (2006) Complications of blood transfusion. *CEACCP*, **6(6):** 225–229.

SBA 36: answer = B – Vaccinations should be given 14 days prior to splenectomy

For elective splenectomies, vaccinations should be given 14 days prior to surgery, as the immune response to the vaccine is thought to be enhanced with an intact spleen. In an emergency splenectomy, vaccinations should be delayed for at least 14 days post-operatively. If the patient has been receiving immunosuppressive therapy, vaccinations should be delayed until 3 months after this has finished.

Gent, L. and Blackie, P. (2017) The spleen. *BJA Education*, **17(6):** 214–220.

SBA 37: answer = A – 2% chlorhexidine gluconate in 10% alcohol spray to skin, air dried

Recommendations from the AAGBI and the NPSA on safe insertion and management of epidurals should be considered. 0.5% chlorhexidine in 70% alcohol is the ideal disinfecting agent for skin. 2% chlorhexidine in 70% alcohol increases the risk of chlorhexidine-related neurotoxicity, and is best avoided. 10% alcohol solutions are not used. Although other answers are also not ideal, they are not imminently threatening.

Bailey, C., Greatorex, B., Hyde, Y. *et al.* (2020) Infection prevention and control guidelines. *AAGBI* [online] DOI http://dx.doi.org/10.21466/g.IPAC2.2020 (accessed 16 February 2022).

Association of Anaesthetists of Great Britain and Ireland; Obstetric Anaesthetists' Association; Regional Anaesthesia UK (2013) Regional anaesthesia and patients with abnormalities of coagulation. *Anaesthesia*, **68:** 966–972.

SBA 38: answer = D – Level with the external auditory meatus

In the sitting position, the arterial transducer should be placed at the level of the external auditory meatus. This will allow cerebral perfusion to be accurately measured. It is also important to maintain normovolaemia at all times during surgery to minimise the risk of venous air embolism.

Jagannathan, S. and Krovvidi, H. (2014) Anaesthetic considerations for posterior fossa surgery. *CEACCP*, **14(5):** 202–206.

SBA 39: answer = E – Severe ventricular aneurysm with thrombus formation

All of the options, with the exception of E, are indications for cardiac transplant. These patients may present either electively or acutely to cardiothoracic theatres for management. They are usually profoundly haemodynamically unstable, and induction should only take place with an experienced cardiac anaesthetist and perfusion team immediately available.

Edwards, S., Allen, S. and Sidebotham, D. (2021) Anaesthesia for heart transplantation. *BJA Education*, **21(8):** 284–291.

SBA 40: answer = A – Phrenic nerve palsy

Phrenic nerve palsy has been noted in up to 100% of ISB done via landmark technique, and those with LA volumes of ≥20ml in various studies. With ultrasound-guided techniques using lower volumes, the incidence is reduced to approximately 50%. This is because the phrenic nerve lies superior to the anterior scalene muscle, and thus is often inadvertently blocked. The incidences of Horner's syndrome and recurrent laryngeal nerve palsy (temporary) are common, but marginally less frequent than phrenic nerve involvement. LA toxicity secondary to systemic absorption and dural puncture are fortunately rare.

Hewson, D., Oldman, M. and Bedforth, N. (2019) Regional anaesthesia for shoulder surgery. *BJA Education*, **19(4):** 98–104.

SBA 41: answer = D – Plasma cholinesterase activity increases from the 10th week of pregnancy

Plasma cholinesterase activity decreases from the 10th week of pregnancy to a maximal reduction by day 3 postpartum. In severe cases this may mean a dose adjustment for succinylcholine, as there may be an increased sensitivity. Oxygen requirements can increase by 60% so patients can quickly become hypoxic – especially considering the FRC is reduced by 30% when in the supine position at term. Progesterone causes a lowering of the CO_2 response threshold, which results in an increase in minute ventilation. The placenta produces ALP at the brush border, so a raised ALP may be a normal finding in the third trimester.

Bedson, R. and Riccoboni, A. (2014) Physiology of pregnancy: clinical anaesthetic implications. *CEACCP*, **14(2):** 69–72.

SBA 42: answer = D – Nasal intubation – size 7

Nasal intubation is required for cosmetic and orthognathic surgery, as assessment of mouth occlusion and the sitting of the 'bite' of the teeth is essential. For most adults, size 7 to 7.5 nasal endotracheal tubes are appropriate.

Beck, J. and Johnston, K. (2014) Anaesthesia for cosmetic and functional maxillofacial surgery. *CEACCP*, **14(1):** 38–42.

SBA 43: answer = C – Peribulbar block

The administration of volume around the orbit, either as local anaesthetic or haematoma, will result in an increase in IOP. This is the case with a peribulbar block. Sub-Tenon's blocks demonstrate a drop in IOP, possibly due to extra-orbital muscle relaxation. The Trendelenburg position (head down) will increase IOP.

Lewis, H. and James, I. (2021) Update on anaesthesia for paediatric ophthalmic surgery. *BJA Education*, **21(1):** 32–38.

Murgatroyd, H. and Bembridge, J. (2008) Intraocular pressure. *CEACCP*, **8(3):** 100–103.

SBA 44: answer = A – Nabiximols (Sativex)

Currently, nabiximols (brand name Sativex) is the only drug directly targeting the endocannabinoid system that is licensed to treat pain in the UK. This is specifically for muscle spasm pain in MS. The other drugs are licensed for treatment of nausea and vomiting, aside from vapourised THC, which is unlicensed for medicinal consumption. Cannabidiol is licensed for paediatric seizure disorders (Lennox–Gastaut syndrome and Dravet syndrome).

NHS (2008) *Medical cannabis (and cannabis oils)*. Available at: www.nhs.uk/conditions/medical-cannabis/ (accessed 18 February 2022).

NICE (2019, updated 2021) *Cannabis-based medicinal products* [NG144]. Available at: www.nice.org.uk/guidance/ng144 (accessed 18 February 2022).

SBA 45: answer = E – There must be an inpatient paediatric facility within the same hospital site if a paediatric list is offered

For paediatric day case surgeries, there does not have to be an inpatient paediatric facility – but there does have to be a robust structure for admitting a patient to a local paediatric unit should the need arise. Ex-premature infants may be safely managed in a day case surgery unit, but there may be the need for additional expertise. Emergency day case surgery can happen with specific procedures (such as peri-anal abscess) and may help to take the pressure away from emergency inpatient resources. There is no upper age limit for day surgery in the national guidelines, but there may be local guidelines in place. Morbidly obese patients can undergo day case surgery, but super-morbidly obese patients should be discussed on a case-by-case basis with the day case surgery lead and parent surgery team.

Quemby, D. and Stocker, M. (2014) Day surgery development and practice: key factors for a successful pathway. *CEACCP*, **14(6):** 256–261.

Royal College of Anaesthetists (2021) *Guidelines for the provision of anaesthesia services for day surgery*. Available at: https://rcoa.ac.uk/gpas/chapter-6 (accessed 15 March 2022).

SBA 46: answer = C – Venous bicarbonate has increased by 2mmol/L in an hour

The aim for the management of diabetic ketoacidosis will be the resolution of the acidosis and control of blood sugar in a timely manner. These patients are commenced on a fixed rate insulin infusion, as well as IV fluids – which in most instances will be 0.9% saline. Key metabolic goals will be the reduction in capillary blood glucose by 3mmol/L in an hour, the increase in bicarbonate by 3mmol/L in an hour, and the reduction in blood ketones by >0.5mmol/L in an hour. If any of these metabolic goals are not met, this should prompt investigation and further management.

Hallett, A., Modi, A. and Levi, N. (2016) Developments in the management of diabetic ketoacidosis in adults: implications for anaesthetists. *BJA Education*, **16(1):** 8–14.

SBA 47: answer = E – 2% hyperbaric prilocaine

Ambulatory surgery refers to patients who can be discharged up to midnight of the day of surgery. Traditionally, spinal techniques have not been performed in the day case surgery setting due to their long duration of action. Although short-acting, lidocaine is contraindicated due to occurrence of transient neurological symptoms (TNS). Hyperbaric bupivacaine can be used, but due to its duration of action it is not commonly used in the ambulatory setting. Prilocaine has been available for use since 2010 and can be used for procedures up to 90 minutes in duration. Its duration of action is short enough to facilitate a same-day discharge. Supplementation of intrathecal analgesia with early oral analgesia means the addition of intrathecal opiates is often unnecessary, and in this case, the history of PONV makes it a relative contraindication.

Rattenberry, W., Hertling, A. and Erskine, R. (2019) Spinal anaesthesia for ambulatory surgery. *BJA Education*, **19(10):** 321–328.

SBA 48: answer = C – ≤100μA

Electrical leakage current is the amount of current that a device loses to its surroundings, and is graded depending on that amount. Type B devices may lose up to 100μA and type C equipment leakage should be below 10μA. There are also type BF and type CF equipment which are within a floating circuit, but the values remain the same.

Singh, S., Ingham, R. and Golding, J. (2011) Basics of electricity for anaesthetists. *CEACCP*, **11(6):** 224–228.

SBA 49: answer = E – Hypofibrinogenaemia is a common finding

AFE occurs in 2 phases, of which phase 2 includes LV failures and DIC. Foetal distress (if before delivery) and hypotension occur in 100% of AFE cases. Tranexamic acid has been shown to reduce mortality in post-partum haemorrhage. Serum C3 and C4 levels have been shown to be low in AFE, but are not significant or specific enough to be diagnostic. Hypofibrinogenaemia is common and requires cryoprecipitate and/or fibrinogen concentrates.

Metodiev, Y., Ramasamy, P. and Tuffnell, D. (2018) Amniotic fluid embolism. *BJA Education*, **18(8):** 234–238.

SBA 50: answer = E – Early administration of steroids

The CRASH trial was a large (around 10 000-patient) randomised controlled trial investigating the use of steroids in traumatic brain injury. The outcome was that steroids should not be used to treat head injury, whatever the severity, due to an increased risk of mortality and morbidity. The other options are all key management goals of the patient with traumatic brain injury to prevent secondary brain injury.

Roberts, I., Yates, D., Sandercock, P. *et al.* (2004) Effect of intravenous corticosteroids on death within 14 days in 10 008 adults with clinically significant head injury (MRC CRASH trial): randomised placebo-controlled trial. *The Lancet*, **364(9442):** 1321–1328.

SBA 51: answer = A – Parietal pleura

The borders of the paravertebral space are:
• Anterior: parietal pleura
• Posterior: superior costotransverse ligament
• Medial: vertebrae, intervertebral foramina
• Lateral: parietal pleura.

Nair, S., Gallagher, H. and Conlon, N. (2020) Paravertebral blocks and novel alternatives. *BJA Education*, **20(5):** 158–165.

SBA 52: answer = A – Fluid restriction

This patient has signs of SIADH, most likely secondary to an underlying diagnosis of small cell lung cancer. The first-line management for SIADH would be fluid restriction, typically to 1L, while further investigation continues. In this case a CT chest / abdomen / pelvis with contrast would be appropriate to screen for the underlying malignancy and spread (staging CT). Demeclocycline and tolvaptan can be used but they are not advised as first-line treatment. Hypertonic saline may be effective in an emergency to raise the sodium levels, but this can also be achieved by fluid restriction. Desmopressin is used in the treatment of diabetes insipidus.

Hirst, C., Allahabadia, A. and Cosgrove, J. (2014) The adult patient with hyponatraemia. *CEACCP*, **15(5):** 248–252.

SBA 53: answer = C – Lack of tongue protrusion

Good airway assessment is imperative to assessing risk and airway management planning. Mouth opening can be impaired by trismus, but lack of tongue protrusion is very sensitive for sublingual involvement and signifies impending airway compromise. Dysphagia and stridor are late signs for airway compromise and stridor may not be present at rest.

Morosan, M., Parbhoo, A. and Curry, N. (2012) Anaesthesia and common oral and maxillo-facial emergencies. *CEACCP*, **2(5):** 257–262.

SBA 54: answer = E – Diclofenac sodium

NSAIDs are best avoided in vascular surgery due to their nephrotoxic potential and risk of exacerbating cardiac disease – which is very common in patients with peripheral arterial disease. Although not contraindicated, tramadol should be used in caution in this population due to the risk of exacerbating delirium.

Fraser, K. and Raju, I. (2015) Anaesthesia for lower limb revascularization surgery. *BJA Education*, **15(5):** 225–230.

SBA 55: answer = B – Superior costotransverse

The superior costotransverse ligament (SCTL) is in continuity with the internal intercostal membrane, and must be pierced to access the paravertebral space. However, as it is a porous structure, it is susceptible to local anaesthetic transfer – as is the case in erector spinae blocks, and other paraspinal techniques.

Nair, S., Gallagher, H. and Conlon, N. (2020) Paravertebral blocks and novel alternatives. *BJA Education*, **20(5):** 158–165.

SBA 56: answer = E – Contact Trust lawyer

The safest option is to contact the Trust lawyer, as it is a very specific case with a complicated ethical dilemma. The patient may be Gillick competent to consent to the surgery but may not be able to refuse the surgery. This is not life or limb surgery so does not need to happen imminently. The patient's parent does not want to re-book the patient at a later date, as there may be issues regarding their ability to care for the patient post-operatively. Administering sedation or proceeding anyway may be seen as assault, as it is clear the patient does not want the surgery. In this instance it is best to contact the Trust lawyer, and although this may take some time, it is the safest from a legal point of view.

Williams, C. and Perkins, R. (2011) Consent issues in children: a law unto themselves? *CEACCP*, **11(3):** 99–103.

SBA 57: answer = A – Cold water immersion

The aim should be to rapidly cool the patient to 39°C and rehydrate them. However, methods which rapidly cool the skin are recommended over body cavity lavage or intravenous cooling catheters. Intravenous fluids do have a place in management, but they should be isotonic or hypertonic and potassium-free wherever possible, as patients tend to be hyperkalaemic. No pharmacological intervention has been shown to be of benefit in exertional heatstroke.

Alexiou, A. and Glazer, J. (2021) Heat stroke in adults. *BMJ Best Practice*. Available at: https://bestpractice.bmj.com/topics/en-gb/3000174 (accessed 18 February 2022).

Grogan, H. and Hopkins, P. (2002) Heat stroke: implications for critical care and anaesthesia. *BJA*, **88(5):** 700–707.

Lipman, G., Gaudio, F., Eifling, K. *et al.* (2019) Wilderness Medicine Society clinical practice guidelines for the prevention and treatment of heat illness: 2019 update. *Wilderness & Environmental Medicine*, **30(S4):** S33–S46.

SBA 58: answer = C – Cannabinoids are a legal additive in the UK

There are currently 4 generations of vaping devices available on the market. Vaping is increasingly common amongst young people and those trying to give up smoking, but the extent of effects on health are not currently known. Vaping devices are known to cause burns and platelet dysfunction.

Cutts, T. and O'Donnell, A. (2021) The implications of vaping for the anaesthetist. *BJA Education*, **21(7):** 243–249.

SBA 59: answer = C – Middle trunk

When there are excessive periods of shoulder depression, such as in steep head-down positioning, there is a risk of injury to the upper and middle trunk. This is further exacerbated by contralateral neck flexion and compression. Injury to the middle trunk gives rise to weakness of shoulder abduction, as well as paraesthesia in the lateral shoulder and arm. The primary nerve affected is the axillary nerve.

Betteridge, N., Taylor, A. and Hartley, R. (2021) Clinical anatomy of the nerve supply to the upper limb. *BJA Education*, **21(12):** 462–471.

SBA 60: answer = B – Cardiorespiratory parameters

In the immediate recovery phase following a general anaesthetic, cardiorespiratory parameters are not considered reliable to assess severity of pain. As a result, their sole use is no longer recommended. Pain scores that are currently advocated for use in the immediate post-operative period include the Pain Assessment in Advanced Dementia Scale (PAINAD), Behavioural Pain Scale (BPS), and the Doloplus-2 pain tool (for cognitively impaired patients). A suitable alternative in patients unable to verbalise includes evaluation of opiate medication requirement.

Small, C. and Laycock, H. (2020) Acute postoperative pain management, *British Journal of Surgery*, **107(2):** e70–80.